Phlebotomy Exam Review

Phlebotomy Exam Review

Ruth E. McCall, MT(ASCP), CLS(NCA)

Director of Phlebotomy Program
Instructor, MLT Program
Albuquerque Technical–Vocational Institute
Albuquerque, New Mexico

Cathee M. Tankersley, MT(ASCP), CLS(NCA)

Director of Phlebotomy, EKG, and EEG Programs
Phoenix College
Phoenix, Arizona

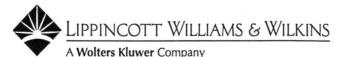

LIPPINCOTT WILLIAMS & WILKINS
A **Wolters Kluwer** Company
Philadelphia · Baltimore · New York · London
Buenos Aires · Hong Kong · Sydney · Tokyo

Acquisitions Editor: *Kathleen P. Lyons*
Project Editor: *Gretchen Metzger*
Production Manager: *Helen Ewan*
Production Coordinator: *Patricia McCloskey*
Design Coordinator: *Melissa Olson*
Indexer: *Anne Cope*

Library of Congress Cataloging-in-Publication Data

McCall, Ruth E.
    Phlebotomy exam review / Ruth E. McCall and Cathee M. Tankersley.
        p.   cm.
    Includes index.
    ISBN 0-397-55232-7 (alk. paper)
    1. Phlebotomy—Examinations, questions, etc.   I. Tankersley, Cathee M.   II. Title
    [DNLM: 1. Phlebotomy—examination questions.   WB 18.2 M4777p 1997]
RB45.15.M332   1997
616.07′561—dc20
DNLM/DLC
for Library of Congress   96-19176
                                                                                                          CIP

The material contained in this volume was submitted as previously unpublished material, except in the instances in which credit has been given to the source from which some of the illustrative material was derived.

Any procedure or practice described in this book should be applied by the health-care practitioner under appropriate supervision in accordance with professional standards of care used with regard to the unique circumstances that apply in each practice situation. Care has been taken to confirm the accuracy of information presented and to describe generally accepted practices. However, the authors, editors, and publisher cannot accept any responsibility for errors or omissions or for any consequences from application of the information in this book and make no warranty, express or implied, with respect to the contents of the book.

The authors and publisher have exerted every effort to ensure that drug selection and dosage set forth in this text are in accordance with current recommendations and practice at the time of publication. However, in view of ongoing research, changes in government regulations, and the constant flow of information relating to drug therapy and drug reactions, the reader is urged to check the package insert for each drug for any change in indications and dosage and for added warnings and precautions. This is particularly important when the recommended agent is a new or infrequently employed drug.

Materials appearing in this book prepared by individuals as part of their official duties as U.S. Government employees are not covered by the above-mentioned copyright.

9   8   7   6   5   4   3   2

To my parents Charles and Marie Ruppert,
my husband John,
and my sons Chris and Scott
for their encouragement, patience,
and support of this effort.

—Ruth E. McCall

To my husband, Tank, and son, Todd,
for their support,
and a special thanks to my daughter, Jaime,
for her contributions and assistance.

—Cathee M. Tankersley

Starting **Phlebotomy Exam Tutor for Windows:**

1. Start up Windows.
2. Insert the **Phlebotomy Exam Tutor** disk into the floppy disk drive.
3. From the Program Manager's File menu, choose the Run command.
4. When the Run dialog box appears, type a:\setup (or b:\setup if you are using the B drive) in the Command Line box. Click OK or press the Enter button.
5. The Phlebotomy Exam Review installation process will begin. A dialog proposing the directory "PER" on the drive containing Windows will appear. If the name and location are correct, click OK. If you want to change this information, type over the existing data then click OK.
6. When the Phlebotomy Exam Review setup routine is complete, a new group called "Phlebotomy Exam Review" will appear on your desktop.
7. Start the Phlebotomy Exam Review by double-clicking on its icon.

PREFACE

Today's phlebotomist is often required to demonstrate competency through national certification. In addition, some states require licensing through competency testing that is independent of national certification. The basic knowledge of phlebotomy theory necessary to pass most of these examinations is similar.

Phlebotomy Exam Review is designed to provide a comprehensive review of current phlebotomy theory and offers an ideal way to study for phlebotomy licensing or national certification exams. It also makes an excellent study guide for students taking formal phlebotomy training programs.

Answering the questions in this review provides the user an opportunity to test his or her knowledge and application of current phlebotomy theory. Theory questions are based on recent National Committee for Clinical Laboratory Standards (NCCLS) guidelines when applicable and are of the standard multiple-choice format used on the national exams. The format of the question unit of the book follows that of the companion textbook, *Phlebotomy Essentials, 2/E* by the same authors. This format makes it easy to locate a topic in the companion textbook if the user is unable to correctly answer a question or wants more information on the topic. This format also makes it an ideal chapter-to-chapter study reference when used in conjunction with the textbook in phlebotomy training programs.

Outstanding features of this book are:

- information on the various exams available, including application fees, format, contact person, and eligibility routes
- a section on study and test-taking skills to help ensure success on the exam
- more than 1000 multiple-choice questions, with correct answers and detailed explanations
- two mock exams, one traditional (pencil and paper) and one computer-based.

This book is designed to help the user identify areas of strength and weakness in his or her phlebotomy knowledge. It is not intended to replace formal education in phlebotomy theory, nor is there any guarantee that using this examination review will ensure passage of any certification or licensing exam.

The authors wish to express their gratitude to all who assisted and supported this effort.

CONTENTS

INTRODUCTION

In today's health care climate, recognition through certification is becoming more popular because of the need for health care professionals to show evidence of proficiency in many different areas of practice.

Certification is evidence that an individual has mastered fundamental competencies in a profession. National Board certification is granted to candidates who have met all the educational or experiential requirements of the agency and have successfully passed the examination.

Presently, five agencies offer certification in phlebotomy. Generally speaking, employers do not favor any single certifying agency, but the applicant may find that one examination better suits his or her needs than another. In making a selection, the applicant may choose from any of the following:

American Medical Technologists
(AMT)
710 Higgins Road
Park Ridge, Illinois 60068
(847) 823-5169
(847) 326-9676 fax

American Society of Clinical
Pathologists (ASCP)
Board of Registry
Lock Box 96215
Chicago, Illinois 60693-6215
(312) 738-1336
(312) 738-1619 fax

American Society of Phlebotomy
Technicians (ASPT)

Post Office Box 1831
Hickory, North Carolina 28603
(704) 322-1334
(704) 326-9676 fax

National Certification Agency for
Medical Laboratory Personnel
(NCA)
Post Office Box 15945-289
Lenexa, Kansas 66285
(913) 438-5110
(913) 541-0156 fax

National Phlebotomy Association, Inc.
(NPA)
5615 Landover Road
Hyattsville, Maryland 20784
(301) 699-3846
(301) 699-5766 fax

All five agencies have examination sites throughout the United States. Two of the agencies also offer examinations in other countries: ASPT in Puerto Rico, Mexico, Canada, and Germany, and NCA in Puerto Rico and Kuwait.

Before 1981, when the National Phlebotomy Association (NPA) offered their first certification exam, national recognition for phlebotomists was unheard of. Since that time more than 60,000 certification exams have been given according to information in the following exam comparison chart. By using the average passing rates between 70% and 80%, it can be estimated that about 45,000 applicants have become certified phlebotomists.

(text continues on page 5)

National Certification Exam Comparisons:

	NPA	ASPT	AMT	NCA	ASCP
Telephone number	(301) 699-3846 (301) 699-5766 (fax)	(704) 322-1334 (704) 326-9676 (fax) (810) 557-4415	(847) 823-5169 (847) 823-0458 (fax)	(913) 438-5110 x453 (913) 541-0156 (fax)	(312) 738-1336 (312) 738-1619 (fax)
Contact	Diane C. Crawford	Ralph & Helen Maxwell Virginia Faber	Cathie Casey	Dede Gish-Panjada	Renne Allegrucci
Date Organization Established	May, 1978	October, 1983	Incorporated, 1939	January, 1977	January, 1928
Examination: Original date given	September, 1981	January, 1984	July, 1992	January, 1985	August, 1989
How often given	Varies with need	On demand	Scheduled throughout the year	Twice a year	Continuously given year round
When given	Schedule 30 days ahead of time	Can give two per day	(see above)	January & July	Monday through Saturday
What days	Whatever specified, except Sunday and holidays	None specified	(see above)	Last Saturday in January & July	Arranged by applicant
Administered by whom	Proctor	Educational directors and lab managers, ASPT representatives	American Medical Technologists proctors	By designees of the testing agency	Sylvan Technology Test Centers
Where	46 states, 73 sites	50 states, numerous sites	At numerous sites	46 states, 75 sites	Most major cities in U.S. & Puerto Rico
Application deadlines	30 days in advance	2 weeks before exam	60 days before scheduled administration	October 1 and April 1	January 2, April 1, July 1, October 2
Fees	$95.00—Includes membership $10.00—Late fee	$45.00 exam fee $25.00 application fee	$59.00 application and examination	$50.00 exam fee	$60.00 exam fee
Exam format	2 parts; 240 questions plus practical portion	220 multiple-choice questions, 20-step practicum	200 multiple-choice questions	100 multiple-choice questions	80 multiple-choice questions given on computer
Based on	Curriculum design for phlebotomy training	ASPT study outline, recognized phlebotomy standards	Phlebotomy technician task delineation (job analysis)	ASCLS phlebotomy performance standards	Board of Registry job analysis

	CPT (NPA)	CPT (ASPT)	RPT (AMT)	CIPlb (NCA)	PBT (ASCP)
Criterion referenced	Yes	Yes	Yes	Yes	Yes
Examination scoring	Hand scored, minimum passing rate: 70% overall	Computer scored, minimum passing rate: 80% overall	Computer scored, scale score 0–100 with 70 or greater equal to passing	Computer scored with minimum passing score for each skill area	Computer scored, scaled score with minimum passing score of 400
Result Report	Letter suggesting review of didactic material	Report gives breakdown in percentages for each area	Scaled score and pass/fail status. Report gives indication which primary content categories exhibited poor performance for candidates who fail.	Report shows score by category with no ranking of applicants.	Scaled score and pass/fail status
Certification Initials	CPT (NPA)	CPT (ASPT)	RPT (AMT)	CIPlb (NCA)	PBT (ASCP)
Grandfathering	*One year continual work experience	Anyone who has passed a national exam, and the ASPT practicum	None	None	None
Recertification	No	Yes	Voluntary continuing educ.—members do not lose certification for noncompliance.	Yes	No
How often	N/A	Every year	N/A	Every 4 yrs by exam or every 2 yrs by cont. ed.	N/A
Routes	N/A	Must have 6.0 contact hours/year	N/A	Retake exam or 4.0 CEUs every 2 years	N/A
Cost	N/A	Retake fee: $25.00	N/A	Reexamination fee: $50.00 Recertification with CEUs: $35.00	Retake fee: $60.00 Allowed only five attempts
Additional Fees	Annual membership fee: $60.00 Late fee: $10.00	Membership fee: $20.00/year Includes newsletter, availability of cont. educ., exam notices, ID card	Membership dues: $44.00/year. Includes newsletters, cont. ed. supplements, ID card, CE report card, & other benefits.	None	Registration fee $25.00/yr Includes journal, ID card, certification renewal seal

(continued)

* Refers to NPA Reclamation Clause used in place of Grandfathering

National Certification Exam Comparisons: (Continued)

	NPA	ASPT	AMT	NCA	ASCP
Eligibility Routes	1. Active phlebotomist with 1 year work experience 2. Student in NPA-approved training program 3. 5.4 CEUs in phlebotomy education if less than 1 year work experience	1. At least 6 months of FT work experience 2. One year PT work experience 3. Completion of an ASPT-approved training program	1. Graduated from an ABHES accredited phlebotomy program 2. Graduate of an acceptable accredited institution's phlebotomy program 3. Completed a phlebotomy training program which includes 120 hrs of didactic & 120 hrs of clinical practicum. 4. Completed 1040 hrs of acceptable work experience within last 3 years	1. Completion of a formal education program 2. One year FT work experience	1. HS diploma or GED and completion of NAACLS-approved program within the last 5 years 2. HS diploma or GED and completion of an acceptable formal structured program with specified curriculum from an accredited institution 3. HS diploma or GED and 1 yr FT acceptable experience within last 5 yrs with specified clinical experience
Other Exams Given by Agency	None	POCT/CLIA waived testing, Blood Donor Specialist, Certified Drug Collection Specialist, EKG Tech., Paramedical Insurance Examiner	MT MLT Registered Medical Assistant (RMA), Registered Dental Assistant (RDA)	CLT, CLS specialists, categoricals, cytogenetics, clinical laboratory director, clinical laboratory supervisor	MLT, MT, specialists, categoricals, histologic technician, histotechnologist, Diplomate in laboratory management
Reciprocity	None	Given in Mexico, Canada, Germany & Puerto Rico	Certificate and licensed phlebotomists	Given in Kuwait & Puerto Rico	None
Continuing Education Offerings	Continuing education mailings to certificate holders and accepts CEUs from NPA sponsored programs and other recognized organizations	National Annual Meeting, Quarterly Regional Seminars, PACE Approved Cross-Training Specialty Programs, Phlebotomy Training Manual available	AMT Step Program and an annual national educational meeting and conference	Offers none, accepts CEUs from professional organizations	National Annual Meeting, regional workshop weeks, and teleconferences
Exams given to date	Over 10,000	Over 21,000	Information not available		Over 10,000

In 1991, the ASCP Board of Registry began administering certification exams by computer. The process used is referred to as "computer adaptive testing". This refined software is programmed to respond to the candidate's pattern of answering the questions by branching from one question to another based on whether the candidate answers it correctly or incorrectly.

Every year increasing numbers of phlebotomists sit for one or more national certification exams, even though most institutions do not require certification as a condition for hire nor is there, in most instances, any remuneration as a result of being certified. Evidence that phlebotomists feel national recognition for competency in their area of expertise is very important to their self-esteem and peer recognition.

The five examinations currently available are based on similar versions of accepted phlebotomy standards of practice. Most often these standards are determined through job/task analysis surveys. Outlines reflecting the exam content and references used in developing the questions are available from all the agencies and will be sent automatically to applicants who apply for the exam.

All five agencies recognize graduation from an approved educational program as a route to be eligible to sit for the exam. Other routes, such as work experience and specific educational requirements are varied depending on the agency. Application deadlines range from 14 days to 90 days and the application can be mailed at any time throughout the year, but will only apply to the offering closest to the date the application is received. The exam formats vary from 80 to 240 questions. An example of an exam's content outline and the percentage of questions in each category is as follows:

NCA CONTENT OUTLINE

1. Health care system—5% recall
   a. identify lab departments
   b. identify departments within health care
   c. identify medical specialties
   d. identify the roles of clinical lab personnel
   e. identify laboratory terminology
2. Infection control—20% recall
   a. identify ways infection is transmitted
      1. airborne
      2. blood/body fluids
      3. contact
   b. practice methods of preventing infection during venipuncture
      1. wear gloves
      2. wear lab coats or other protective garments
      3. wear masks, face shields, goggles when warranted
      4. wash hands and change gloves between venipuncture
      5. dispose of sharps
   c. ensure proper infection control within lab setting
      1. recognize clean and contaminated areas
      2. remove and dispose of gowns, lab coats, when leaving contaminated areas for clean areas
      3. wear protective clothing and equipment when processing specimens
      4. disinfect all work surfaces at least once per shift
      5. dispose of lab specimens in biohazard containers
      6. use spill kits for biohazardous spills
3. Safety—20% recall
   a. practice institution procedures for the following:
      1. fire safety
      2. natural disasters
      3. hazardous materials
      4. general physical safety
      5. patient first aid
   b. recognize regulatory agencies, CDC, OSHA, etc.
4. Anatomy and physiology of body systems—5% recall
   a. recognize anatomic regions
   b. recognize the components of circulatory system

1. blood (rbc, wbc, plasma, serum)
2. heart (anatomy, function)
3. blood vessels (arteries, veins, capillaries)

5. Importance of specimen collection—35% recall
   a. ensure proper collection for specimen integrity
      1. collect proper sample for test ordered
      2. meet specimen requirements (fasting, time considerations, temperature, order of draw)
      3. use proper technique
      4. use appropriate site for collection (coagulation testing)
      5. label specimens following laboratory protocol
   b. ensure proper patient identification
   c. collection equipment
      1. list equipment needed for collection of blood specimens by venipuncture
      2. list equipment needed for collection of blood by skin puncture
      3. list equipment needed for special blood collection (blood culture, blood gases, bleeding times)
      4. recognize the various types of additives used in blood collections and identify their uses
   d. specimen requisition, transport, and processing
      1. use specimen information systems
      2. recognize information required on lab requisitions
      3. recognize primary information required on lab specimens (patient name, date/time collected, ID)
      4. employ transport systems
      5. transport tests that require special handling
      6. ensure safety while transporting specimens
      7. ensure proper specimen processing
6. Quality assurance—4% recall, 6% application

   a. recognize lab's quality assurance markets (specimen collection, specimen transport, patient preparation and identification)
   b. ensure all requirements for specimen quality have been met (correct specimen collected, proper venipuncture technique used, proper transport of sample has been employed)
   c. attend continuing education and inservice training, as required
7. Communication—2% recall, 3% application
   a. use professionalism when communicating with patient, staff, and visitors
   b. recognize the patient's bill of rights
   c. use positive body language (smiling, good grooming, eye contact)
   d. maintain patient confidentiality at all times

STUDYING AND TEST-TAKING TIPS

Regardless of the type of test you are preparing for, there are numerous techniques that you can use to study and review effectively and improve your test-taking ability. The following information is designed to help you develop a study plan, control the study and test-taking environment, and learn key ways to retain information while studying. The desired result is to be able to effectively express your knowledge of a subject while taking a test.

HOW TO PREPARE TO STUDY

Cultivate a Positive Attitude

The old adage, "You can do anything if you set your mind to it," makes a lot of sense. Those who think they can succeed at something and have a plan to achieve it are usually successful. Those who think they will fail usually do. If your goal is to pass a national certification exam, your belief that you will be able to successfully pass that exam actually helps you achieve that goal. In addition, your attitude plays an important role in determining how you approach preparation for an exam and ultimately how well you do on the actual exam. A positive attitude during the study process will result in more effective studying and increase learning and retention. Bringing a positive attitude to the test will help relieve the stress associated with the testing process and leave your mind free to think logically and make you a more successful test taker.

Plan to Study

A key element of effective studying is your ability to manage your study or review time. Plan to study. Develop a routine by establishing a particular time and place to study. Committing yourself to a regular routine eliminates the continual need to decide when and where to study. This keeps you in control and helps eliminate procrastination.

Establish a Consistent Study Setting

Choose a site that is compatible with study activities, such as a desk or table. Make sure the site is comfortable and has adequate lighting to minimize eye strain and fatigue. Resist the temptation to get too comfortable, however. Avoid beds or couches where you may become too relaxed and doze off.

Limit Distractions

Select a place to study where you are less likely to be disturbed by family members, room-mates, pets, TV, phones etc.

Do not answer the phone. If you do not have an answering machine, unplug the phone.

Limit Commitments

Do not disrupt your study schedule unless it's really important. Learn to say "no." Put a "Do Not Disturb" sign on the door.

WHEN TO STUDY

Study When You are Rested

You are more alert when you are rested. Do not study when you are already physically or emotionally tired, and never study to the point of exhaustion.

Follow Your Daily Biorhythm

If possible, study during a time of day when you are most alert and efficient. For example, if you are a morning person, try to arrange study time in the morning.

HOW TO STUDY

Have a Review Strategy

Decide in advance how you will review the material and allow adequate time to accomplish everything you want to do. Use whatever method works best for you.

Effective study strategies include reviewing your notes, textbook, and study questions, and taking practice tests or mock exams.

Consider Forming a Study Group

Set aside some time to study with other students or peers who are also preparing to take the same exam. Members of study groups tend to motivate each other. Members can also share study tips and techniques that work well for them.

Establish a Realistic Study Schedule

Avoid resorting to marathon study sessions. Short 1- to 3-hour study sessions on a regular basis are usually more beneficial than an occasional long drawn-out session.

Use Time Effectively

Copy information that needs to be memorized into a small notebook or on note cards and carry them with you. That way you can study small amounts while waiting in line, riding the bus, or waiting for appointments. Note cards can also be taped on mirrors, cupboards, etc. for quick reviews in between other chores or activities.

Take Breaks

Don't forget the old saying "All work and no play makes Jack a dull boy." You by no means want to be "dull" on test day. Schedule breaks into your allotted study time. The ideal break should be short enough to relieve stress but not so extended that you lose focus, interest, or rhythm.

Watch The Time

Keep track of the time and don't waste it. If you get frustrated or your attention starts to wander, take a break.

WHAT TO STUDY

Study difficult or boring concepts or topics first.

Don't Try to Study Everything at Once

Think about the answer to the joke, "How do you eat an elephant?" Answer: "One bite at a time!" Divide extensive topics into smaller portions.

Study What is Appropriate

Try not to overstudy or do more than necessary. Don't repeatedly go over material you already know. Review it every so often to make certain you still remember it, but don't spend a lot of time on it. For example, it would be a waste of time to read the textbook or your class notes over and over. A more effective method would be to review your notes and refer to the textbook to clarify concepts or information you have forgotten or do not completely understand.

Use the Exam Review Effectively

Once you feel that you are familiar with the material, try to answer the questions from this exam review. Refer to the textbook for information if you can't answer a question or still need to clarify material after you read the explanation for the correct answer.

Take the Mock Exams

When you feel you have a good grasp of the material, you are ready to take the mock exams. Again, refer to the text or class notes when you can't answer a question. Never attempt to memorize questions and answers. The intent of the study questions and mock exams is to help you identify areas in which you are weak. In addition, taking the computer mock exam will help you feel more comfortable taking a computer exam in the future.

HOW TO IMPROVE YOUR THINKING SKILLS

Multiple-choice questions usually cover six commonly recognized thinking levels. From lowest to highest they are: memory, comprehension, application, analysis, synthesis, and evaluation. When studying for multiple-choice tests, many students mistakenly spend their study time learning at the lowest level, memorizing facts without understanding how to analyze and apply the information. Learning how to identify the various thinking levels and using the skills associated with them as you study should help to enhance your knowledge of the subject and help you be a successful test-taker.

Memory Skills

Memory questions require the lowest level of thinking and involve the ability to recall specific information such as terminology, structures, classifications, facts, or concepts. Information of this type is most commonly memorized using techniques involving constant repetition. Examples of memorization techniques include reciting information aloud, listing information, and using flash cards. Information learned this way is committed to short-term memory and may be forgotten unless reinforced using other study methods or practical application.

The following are ways to assist in the memorization of information and enhance recall.

ABCs

Associating information with letters of the alphabet is an effective means of recalling information. Each letter of the alphabet acts as a cue or hint to recall information. You can make up your own ABCs to remember information as well as use established ones such as:

The ABCs of cardiopulmonary resuscitation are: A = airway, open the airway; B = breathing, perform rescue breathing; and C = circulation, initiate chest compressions.

Acronyms

Another helpful technique used to recall information is the use of acronyms or words formed by the first letter of a series of statements or facts. Each letter of the word is a memory jog to recall previously learned information.

An example is the acronym RACE used to remember action to take in the event of a fire. R = rescue; A = alarm; C = confine; E = extinguish.

Acrostics

Acrostics are catchy phrases or jingles where the first letter of each word helps you to remember certain information. An example is the jingle used to help remember the order of draw for the evacuated tube method of venipuncture. Stop, red light, green light, go. S = sterile tubes, R = red or SSTs, L = light blue, G = green, L = lavender, G = gray.

Imaging

Forming a mental picture associated with the information is another technique used to recall information. For example one way to remember that a lipemic specimen is caused by fatty substances in the blood that make the serum appear cloudy or milky looking is to visualize a fat, white cloud when thinking or saying the term lipemic.

Comprehension Skills

Comprehension questions test your ability to understand information. To answer comprehension questions you must not only recall information, but you must also be able to understand the significance of the information. Comprehension questions test your ability to interpret information to draw conclusions or determine consequences, effects, or implications. A good way to enhance comprehension of material is to ask yourself what is the significance of this information—"how" or "why" is this information useful? Again, using the term "lipemic" as an example, once we know what the term lipemic means and what a lipemic specimen looks like, we can now ask ourself "What is the significance of a lipemic specimen? Why or how is this information useful?" One answer is that a lipemic specimen is a clue that the patient was not fasting. This is significant if the test was ordered fasting. Lipemia also interferes with the testing process for some chemistry tests. Now we not only can recall facts, we are learning to comprehend the significance of these facts.

Application Skills

Application questions test your ability to use information. Answering application questions requires that you not only remember and comprehend information, but that you are able to relate that information to a real-life situation. Again, using the example of the term lipemic, an application question might be:

When processing a specimen for a fasting glucose test, you notice that the specimen is lipemic. What does this tell you about the specimen?

Thought process: Lipemia can occur after eating fatty foods. If the specimen is lipemic the patient must have eaten recently, which means the specimen is probably not a fasting specimen.

Analysis Skills

Analysis questions test your ability to analyze or evaluate information. Analysis questions often require you to evaluate several options to reach an answer. You must be able to recognize differences and determine the significance of several choices before arriving at your answer.

Example: Which of the following specimens would most likely be rejected for testing?

a. lipemic specimen submitted for glucose testing
b. platelet count collected in an EDTA tube
c. routine UA in an unsterile container
d. specimen for potassium testing that is hemolyzed

The following is a typical thought process used to analyze the choices to the question above and determine the correct answer:

A lipemic specimen is an indication that the patient was not fasting, but it doesn't say it was a fasting glucose. In addition, a few people have lipemic serum for other reasons, so the specimen would not necessarily be rejected.

A platelet count **should** be collected in EDTA, so it wouldn't be rejected.

A urine C&S must be collected in a sterile container, but a routine UA **doesn't have to be,** so it wouldn't be rejected.

Lastly, hemolysis liberates potassium from the red blood cells. That means a hemolyzed potassium specimen will yield erroneous results. A hemolyzed potassium specimen would most likely be rejected. The answer has to be "d."

HOW TO ANSWER MULTIPLE-CHOICE QUESTIONS

For written examinations, jot down memory aids in the margins if you are allowed.
Read the question carefully.
Do not assume information that is not given.
Eliminate choices that are clearly incorrect.
Answer the easy questions first.
Don't spend a lot of time on questions you can't answer.

If you don't know the answer, skip the question and come back later. Information in other questions may remind you of the correct answer. If you still do not know the answer, try to make an educated guess.

Do not change answers without a good reason. Your first guess is usually your best unless other questions remind you of the correct response.

TIPS FOR TEST DAY

Get a good night's sleep before the test.

Collect the items that you must bring to the test, such as identification and test documents, ID, calculator, pencils, etc., ahead of time so that you won't be scrambling to find them at the last minute.

Wear comfortable clothes to the exam. Dress in layers so that you can adapt in case the room is too cold or too warm.

Know your test site. If the test is in a location that you are not familiar with, drive by the testing site a day or two before the exam. If possible travel during the same time frame as when you will be traveling to the actual test. Allow yourself extra travel time the day of the test in case there are unexpected delays.

Arrive early for the test. That way you can get yourself situated and mentally prepared. You also have the opportunity to situate yourself in a location that is comfortable to you and suits your needs, rather than having to quickly choose from the seats that are left.

Listen carefully while test directions are given. Ask for clarification from the proctor if you do not understand something.

Try to relax. Pause to take a deep breath and stretch now and then.

OVERCOMING TEST ANXIETY

Being well-prepared is an excellent way to reduce test anxiety. Familiarity with the material builds confidence. The more familiar you are with the material, the more confident you will be. The more confident you are, the better you will do on the exam. Confidence in your ability and a positive attitude about your chances of success go a long way toward relieving stress or anxiety towards the testing process.

Exam Review

I

Introduction to Phlebotomy

REVIEW QUESTIONS

1. An agency that certifies phlebotomists?
   a. American Society of Clinical Pathologists (ASCP)
   b. Joint Committee for Accrediting Healthcare Organizations (JCAHO)
   c. National Accrediting Agency for Clinical Laboratory Sciences (NAACLS)
   d. National Committee for Clinical Laboratory Standards (NCCLS)

2. An agency that has an approval process for phlebotomy programs?
   a. JCAHO
   b. NAACLS
   c. National Certification Agency for Medical Laboratory Personnel (NCA)
   d. NCCLS

15

3. Drawing a patient's blood without his or her permission can result in a charge of:
   a. assault and battery
   b. invasion of privacy
   c. malpractice
   d. negligence

4. What does the term "tort" mean?
   a. a criminal action
   b. monetary award
   c. personal injury or malpractice
   d. wrongful act resulting in injury or damage

5. The *primary* duty of a phlebotomist:
   a. accession specimens
   b. collect blood specimens
   c. collect skin puncture specimens
   d. process specimens

6. Promoting good public relations is a part of the phlebotomist's role because:
   a. a phlebotomist is a representative of the laboratory
   b. good public relations promotes a harmonious relationship with visitors, staff, and patients.
   c. the patient often equates blood-drawing experiences with the caliber of overall care received while in the hospital
   d. all of the above

7. Two phlebotomists are discussing a patient's condition in the elevator. They are overheard by the patient's daughter. This is an example of:
   a. failure to exercise reasonable care
   b. improper or unskilled care
   c. invasion of privacy
   d. mistreatment of a patient

8. Which is *not* a step in risk management?
   a. breach of confidentiality
   b. education of employees and patients
   c. identification of risk
   d. treatment of risk using procedures already in place

9. *"Primum non nocere"* comes from the Hippocratic Oath and means:
   a. first do no harm
   b. first things first
   c. quality is foremost
   d. ready to serve

10. Which of the following is *not* an example of good work ethics?
    a. accountability
    b. dependability
    c. liability
    d. reliability

11. Phlebotomy is used as a therapeutic treatment for:
    a. diabetes
    b. hypothyroidism
    c. phlebitis
    d. polycythemia

12. Which of the following would *not* violate a patient's right to confidentiality?
    a. indicating the nature of a patient's disease on the door
    b. keeping a list of human immunodeficiency virus (HIV)– positive patients posted in the laboratory
    c. posting a patient's laboratory results on a bulletin board in his or her room
    d. sharing collection site information on a difficult patient

13. Which is *not* a reason for the phlebotomist to participate in continuing education programs? To:
    a. follow Centers for Disease Control (CDC) mandates
    b. learn new techniques
    c. remain current in phlebotomy technology
    d. renew certification

14. Unauthorized release of confidential patient information is called:
    a. assault and battery
    b. invasion of privacy
    c. negligence
    d. violation of informed consent

15. Civil law involves:
    a. crimes against the state
    b. laws established by governments
    c. offenses for which a person may be imprisoned
    d. tort actions between private parties
16. Recognition by one organization of a certification granted by another is called:
    a. accreditation
    b. liability
    c. licensure
    d. reciprocity
17. The term "phlebotomy" is derived from Greek words that literally translated mean to:
    a. cut a vein
    b. draw blood
    c. stick a vein
    d. suck blood
18. Which of the following is *not* a phlebotomist's duty?
    a. collect blood specimens
    b. perform laboratory computer operations
    c. start intravenous lines (IVs)
    d. transport specimens to the laboratory
19. What are the credentials of an NCA-certified phlebotomist?
    a. RPT
    b. CLPlb
    c. CPT
    d. PBT
20. Which of the following ancient bloodletting instruments has its modern day counterpart in bleeding time devices?
    a. bleeding bowl
    b. fleam
    c. scarificator
    d. syringe
21. Malpractice is a claim of:
    a. assault and battery
    b. breach of confidentiality
    c. improper treatment
    d. invasion of privacy
22. Proof of participation in workshops to upgrade skills required by some agencies in order to renew certification is called:
    a. accreditation
    b. continuing education units (CEUs)
    c. essentials
    d. reciprocity
23. Which organization provides voluntary laboratory inspections and proficiency testing?
    a. College of American Pathologists (CAP)
    b. JCAHO
    c. NCA
    d. Occupational Safety and Health Administration (OSHA)
24. Which is *not* an example of negligence? The phlebotomist fails to:
    a. return a bedrail to the upright position
    b. put a needle in the sharps container
    c. report significant changes in patient condition
    d. obtain a specimen from a combative patient
25. A national organization that sets standards for phlebotomy procedures.
    a. ASCP
    b. NAACLS
    c. NCA
    d. NCCLS
26. Which of the following is *not* a "patient right"? The right to:
    a. a complete explanation of his or her bill
    b. confidentiality of his or her records
    c. refuse treatment
    d. know the medical status of his or her health providers

ANSWERS TO REVIEW QUESTIONS

1. *a.* ASCP is one of five national organizations that certify phlebotomists. Certification is a process that indicates the completion of defined academic and training requirements and the attainment of a satisfactory score on a national examination.

2. *b.* NAACLS is one of the agencies that approves phlebotomy programs. The approval process is similar to accreditation; however, there is no on-site survey.

3. *a.* Assault is defined as the threat to touch a person. Actually touching a person without his or her consent is called battery. If a patient refuses to give his or her permission or consent for blood to be drawn and a phlebotomist continues with the procedure, the phlebotomist can be charged with assault and battery.

4. *d.* A "tort" is a wrongful act for which a civil action can be brought. A claim of malpractice, or in other words, a wrongful act resulting in injury, is only one example of a tort action.

5. *b.* Many duties fall under the role of a phlebotomist, but the primary one is to collect a quality blood specimen.

6. *d.* All of the above is the correct answer because as a "public relations officer" everything the phlebotomist does reflects on the whole facility.

7. *c.* Phlebotomists must be careful not to discuss patient information where they might be overheard. Not only is this considered unprofessional, but it is also considered unauthorized release of patient information and the phlebotomist could face a charge of invasion of privacy.

8. *a.* Risk management involves careful planning in the form of an established procedure and designated steps. Breach of confidentiality caused by the unauthorized release of information concerning a patient can lead to the implementation of risk management techniques.

9. *a.* The primary objective in any health care professional's code of ethics must always be the patient's welfare, "first, do no harm."

10. *c.* Good work ethics include accountability, dependability, and reliability. Liability, defined as an obligation to make good any loss or damage that occurs in a transaction, is invoked when malpractice occurs.

11. *d.* Polycythemia is a condition caused by overproduction of red blood cells and therapy consists of removing some of the blood followed by chemotherapy.

12. *d.* As a professional, the phlebotomist should recognize that *all* patient information, such as disease status and laboratory results, is absolutely private or confidential.

13. *a.* Continuing education for a health professional should support the growth of knowledge in the increasingly complex field of health care. Proof of continuing education is necessary for a phlebotomist to recertify by the NCA. The CDC is not involved in continuing education or recertification.

14. *b.* Unauthorized release of confidential patient information is called "invasion of privacy" and can result in a civil lawsuit.

15. *d.* Civil law is defined as the body of law having to do with private rights of individuals, and "tort" is a wrongful act for which a civil action can be brought. For example, a claim of malpractice because of harm or injury to a patient by a phlebotomist is a civil wrong or tort.

16. *d.* Reciprocity or recognition of a license or certificate from one state to another may be granted to a professional who moves from one state to another.

17. *a.* Literal translation of the word phlebotomy comes from the Greek words "phlebos" meaning vein and "tome" meaning incision or to make an incision (cut) in a vein.

18. *c.* With the advent of multiskilling in the health care field phlebotomists duties are expanding; however, starting IVs is not within the phlebotomist's scope of practice at this time. Nursing assistant duties along with specimen processing and point-of-care testing are fast becoming part of the job description of the phlebotomist.

19. *b.* Each certifying agency awards a designated title and initials to phlebotomists who successfully pass the national examination. NCA has chosen the initials CLPlb (NCA) to designate the title of Clinical Laboratory Phlebotomist.

20. *c.* A scarificator (Fig. 1-1) had several crescent-shaped, spring-loaded blades concealed within a boxlike case which, when activated, made several cuts parallel to each other. Lancets were called fleams and were used to slice a vein, the specimen was collected in a "bleeding bowl."

21. *c.* Malpractice can be described as improper or negligent treatment resulting in injury, loss, or damage for which a malpractice claim can be filed.

22. *b.* A number of organizations sponsor workshops and seminars to enable phlebotomists and other health care workers to earn credit required to renew certification. Credits (in the form of certificates) awarded on completion of these events are called continuing education units (CEUs). Copies of these certificates can be sent to certifying agencies as "proof of continuing education."

23. *a.* College of American Pathologists (CAP), is a national organization

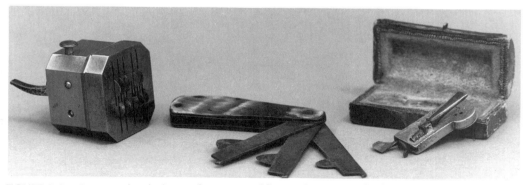

FIGURE 1-1. Octagonal multiple scarificator, set of fleams (lancets), and schnapper with leather-covered wooden case. (Courtesy Robert Kravetz, MD, FACP, FACG, Phoenix, AZ.)

whose members are board-certified pathologists. Services offered by CAP include laboratory inspection and proficiency testing.

24. *d.* Forgetting to return a bedrail to its upright position, failure to discard needles properly (such as dropping them in the trash instead of the sharps container), and not reporting an obvious problem with a patient's condition such as severe breathing difficulties or inability to awaken could all lead to serious consequences and are examples of negligence or failure to exercise reasonable care. Failing to obtain a specimen from a patient is not negligence. Collecting a specimen from a combative patient against his or her will could be considered assault and battery.

25. *d.* The NCCLS develops guidelines and sets standards of performance for all areas of the clinical laboratory. These guidelines are often the basis of approval standards and certification examination questions.

26. *d.* According to the Patient's Bill of Rights, a medical institution has a responsibility to recognize certain established rights of a patient. However, patients do not have the right to know the personal medical history of their nurse or doctor.

The Health Care Setting

A. **Types of Health Care**
   1. *Inpatient/Tertiary Care*
   2. *Outpatient/Ambulatory Care*
     a. *Primary/Physician's Office Laboratory (POLs)*
     b. *Secondary*
   3. *Public Health Services*

B. **Financing**
   1. *Third-Party Payers*
     a. *Types of Coverage*
     b. *Methods of Payment*
     c. *PPS and Diagnostic-Related Groups (DRGs)*
     d. *Accepting Assignment*
     e. *Cost Shifting*
     f. *Capitation*
   2. *Insurance Based on Employment*
     a. *Voluntary Health Insurance*
     b. *Managed Care*
       (1) *Health Maintenance Organizations (HMOs)*
       (2) *Preferred Provider Organizations (PPOs)*
     c. *Social Insurance Programs/ Entitlements*
       (1) *Workers' Compensation*
       (2) *Medicare*
     d. *Public Welfare*
       (1) *Medicaid*
       (2) *Arizona Health Care Cost Containment System (AHCCCS)*
   3. *The Changing Health Care System*

C. **Medical Specialties**
   1. *Dermatology*
   2. *Endocrinology*
   3. *Family Practice*
   4. *Gastroenterology*
   5. *Geriatrics*
   6. *Gerontology*
   7. *Hematology*
   8. *Internal Medicine*
   9. *Neonatology*
   10. *Neurology*
   11. *Obstetrics/Gynecology*
   12. *Oncology*
   13. *Ophthalmology*
   14. *Orthopedics*
   15. *Pediatrics*
   16. *Urology*

D. **Hospital Organization**
   1. *Departments Within the Hospital*
     a. *Patient Care Services*
       (1) *Nursing*
       (2) *Emergency Room(ER)/ Emergency Department (ED)*
       (3) *Intensive Care Unit (ICU)*
     b. *Support Services*
       (1) *Central Supply*
       (2) *Dietary*
       (3) *Environmental Services*
       (4) *Health Information Technology*
     c. *Professional Services*
       (1) *Cardiodiagnostics/ Electrocardiography (ECG/EKG)*
       (2) *Clinical Laboratory*
       (3) *Electroneurodiagnostics/ Electroencephalography (EEG)*
       (4) *Occupational Therapy (OT)*
       (5) *Pharmacy*
       (6) *Physical Therapy (PT)*
       (7) *Respiratory Therapy (RT)*
       (8) *Radiology*
     d. *Clinical Laboratory Services*
       (1) *Specimen Collection Services*

(2) *Specimen Processing and Handling*
   (a) *Onsite*
   (b) *Offsite/Referencing*
(3) *Clinical Analysis Area*
   (a) *Hematology*
   (b) *Coagulation*
   (c) *Urinalysis*
   (d) *Microbiology*
   (e) *Chemistry*
   (f) *Serology/Immunology*
   (g) *Blood Bank/ Immunohematology*
(4) *Anatomic and Surgical Pathology*
   (a) *Histology*
   (b) *Cytology*
   (c) *Cytogenetics*
(5) *Point-of-Care Testing (POCT)*

e. *Support Services*
   (1) *Education*
   (2) *Outreach Programs*
E. **Clinical Laboratory Personnel**
   1. *Laboratory Director/Pathologist*
   2. *Laboratory Administration/ Laboratory Manager*
   3. *Technical Supervisors*
   4. *Medical Technologist/Clinical Laboratory Scientist*
   5. *Medical Laboratory Technicians/ Clinical Laboratory Technicians*
   6. *Phlebotomist*
F. **Clinical Laboratory Personnel**
   1. *Director*
   2. *Technical Consultant*
   3. *Clinical Consultant*
   4. *Testing Personnel*
   5. *General Supervisor*

REVIEW QUESTIONS

1. Which laboratory department performs tests to identify abnormalities of the blood and blood-forming tissues?
   a. chemistry
   b. hematology
   c. microbiology
   d. urinalysis

2. Another term for outpatient care is:
   a. ambulatory care
   b. nonambulatory care
   c. nursing home care
   d. rehabilitation care

3. Radioimmunoassay would most likely be performed in:
   a. coagulation
   b. hematology
   c. immunology
   d. special chemistry

4. Complete patient medical history records are maintained by:

   a. central supply
   b. environmental services
   c. health information technology
   d. nursing

5. Which of the following tests would be performed in surgical pathology?
   a. compatibility testing
   b. enzyme immunoassay
   c. frozen section
   d. triglycerides

6. Diagnosis and treatment of joint and muscle diseases is part of which medical specialty?
   a. dermatology
   b. gastroenterology
   c. internal medicine
   d. rheumatology

7. Which laboratory department would perform glucose testing?
   a. chemistry

b. coagulation
c. cytology
d. hematology

8. Which of the following tests is performed in the coagulation department?
   a. blood urea nitrogen (BUN)
   b. complete blood count (CBC)
   c. glucose
   d. protime (PT)

9. Which laboratory worker has a bachelor's degree, or equivalent, in medical technology?
   a. clinical laboratory scientist (CLS)
   b. clinical laboratory technician (CLT)
   c. medical laboratory technician (MLT)
   d. Phlebotomy Technician (PBT)

10. The medical specialty that treats skeletal system disorders:
    a. gastroenterology
    b. neurology
    c. orthopedics
    d. pediatrics

11. Another name for blood bank is:
    a. immunohematology
    b. immunology
    c. microbiology
    d. serology

12. Hospitals referred to as "community hospitals" are usually:
    a. federal hospitals
    b. investor-owned hospitals
    c. nongovernment, nonprofit hospitals
    d. state hospitals

13. With which other hospital department would the laboratory coordinate therapeutic drug monitoring?
    a. nuclear medicine
    b. pharmacy
    c. physical therapy
    d. radiology

14. Which department processes and stains tissue samples for microscopic analysis?
    a. chemistry
    b. coagulation

c. histology
d. microbiology

15. Which of the following personnel is *not* required to have a college degree or equivalent?
    a. clinical laboratory scientist
    b. medical technologist
    c. phlebotomist
    d. none of the above

16. An appendectomy performed in a freestanding ambulatory surgical center is an example of:
    a. managed care
    b. primary care
    c. secondary care
    d. tertiary care

17. What department would perform blood cultures?
    a. chemistry
    b. hematology
    c. microbiology
    d. urinalysis

18. Electrolyte testing includes:
    a. bilirubin, creatinine
    b. BUN, cholesterol
    c. glucose, uric acid
    d. sodium, potassium

19. What is the responsibility of a clinical consultant under the Clinical Laboratory Improvement Ammendments of 1988 (CLIA '88)?
    a. oversees the entire operation of the laboratory
    b. provides direct supervision to testing personnel
    c. is responsible for technical aspects of the laboratory
    d. serves as a liaison between the laboratory and its clients

20. An SMAC would be performed in:
    a. chemistry
    b. hematology
    c. histology
    d. microbiology

21. Which laboratory department performs chromosome studies?
    a. chemistry
    b. coagulation
    c. cytogenetics
    d. hematology

22. Global capitation is defined as:
    a. annual rate adjustments by Medicare
    b. fee for service based on the going rate
    c. retrospective reimbursement of services
    d. all of the above

23. A mechanism that pays a health care provider a set fee regardless of the volume of services is called:
    a. capitation
    b. entitlement
    c. cost shifting
    d. fee for service

24. Prepaid group health care organizations in which members pay flat fees for defined services are called:
    a. DRGs
    b. HMOs
    c. PPGs
    d. PPOs

25. Which department is responsible for administering a patient's oxygen therapy?
    a. cardiodiagnostics
    b. electroencephalography
    c. physical therapy
    d. respiratory therapy

26. Which hospital department performs diagnostic tests and monitors therapy of heart patients?
    a. EEG
    b. EKG
    c. ER
    d. ICU

27. A direct antibody test (Coombs) is performed in:
    a. hematology
    b. immunohematology
    c. immunology
    d. urinalysis

28. Which of the following titles is equivalent to medical laboratory technician?
    a. CLS
    b. CLT
    c. laboratory assistant
    d. phlebotomist

29. A hospital department that gives increased bedside care for patients in medically fragile condition:
    a. ECG
    b. EEG
    c. ER
    d. ICU

30. Public health agencies function at which level of government?
    a. federal
    b. local
    c. state
    d. all of the above

31. A laboratory department that tests specimens for the presence of bacteria:
    a. chemistry
    b. hematology
    c. microbiology
    d. serology

32. The term used to describe sophisticated and highly complex medical care is:
    a. managed care
    b. primary care
    c. secondary care
    d. tertiary care

33. A patient in labor would normally be admitted to which of the following medical specialty departments?
    a. cardiodiagnostics
    b. geriatrics
    c. obstetrics
    d. pediatrics

34. A function of radiation therapy is:
    a. administration of oxygen therapy
    b. brain wave mapping and polysomnography

c. imaging by means of x-rays

d. treating cancer using high-energy x-rays

35. Toxicology is often a part of which of the following laboratory departments?
    a. chemistry
    b. coagulation
    c. hematology
    d. urinalysis

36. A physician who is a specialist in diagnosing disease from laboratory findings:
    a. administrative technologist
    b. laboratory director
    c. medical technologist
    d. pathologist

37. Which of the following is a hematology test?
    a. C & S
    b. CBC
    c. CSF
    d. SMAC

38. The department that injects patients with radioactive dyes that can interfere with laboratory testing is:
    a. electroneurodiagnostics
    b. nuclear medicine
    c. pharmacy
    d. respiratory therapy

39. Which department performs carcinoembryonic antigen (CEA) testing?
    a. chemistry
    b. hematology
    c. microbiology
    d. serology

40. Which department performs x-ray procedures and other imaging techniques to aid in diagnosis?
    a. occupational therapy
    b. pharmacy
    c. radiology
    d. respiratory therapy

41. Which of the following is an example of an inpatient care facility?

    a. day-surgery facility
    b. dentist's office
    c. hospital
    d. physician's office

42. Which of the following would most likely be performed in the serology department?
    a. BUN
    b. CBC
    c. PT
    d. rapid plasma reagin (RPR)

43. Which of the following laboratory personnel has the same qualifications as a medical technologist?
    a. clinical laboratory technician
    b. clinical laboratory scientist
    c. medical laboratory technician
    d. pathologist

44. Which department would perform a hemogram?
    a. chemistry
    b. hematology
    c. immunohematology
    d. immunology

45. This department may examine specimens microscopically for the presence of crystals, casts, bacteria, and blood cells:
    a. chemistry
    b. hematology
    c. microbiology
    d. urinalysis

46. This hospital department provides therapy to restore patient mobility.
    a. cardiodiagnostics
    b. physical therapy
    c. radiology
    d. respiratory therapy

47. Brain wave mapping and evoked potential is performed by:
    a. ECG
    b. EEG
    c. OT
    d. RT

48. Which of the following statements is *not* the primary objective of managed care? To:
    a. enhance cost containment
    b. facilitate the management of patient needs
    c. increase revenue from services offered
    d. maintain quality care

49. A new category of personnel that works as part of the nursing team, performing nursing and phlebotomy duties along with ancillary testing.
    a. associate's degree nurse (ADN)
    b. certified nursing assistant (CNA)
    c. emergency medical technician (EMT)
    d. patient care technician (PCT)

50. Which medical specialty treats patients with tumors?
    a. geriatrics
    b. oncology
    c. ophthalmology
    d. orthopedics

51. Which of the following laboratory personnel has an associate's degree or equivalent?
    a. clinical laboratory scientist
    b. clinical laboratory technician
    c. medical technologist
    d. phlebotomist

52. A specimen for ova and parasite testing would be sent to:
    a. chemistry
    b. coagulation
    c. microbiology
    d. urinalysis

53. The process of identifying an organism and determining the appropriate antibiotic for treatment is called;
    a. antibody screening
    b. C & S testing
    c. microscopic analysis
    d. radioimmunoassay

54. When a health care provider agrees with a private insurer to accept a fixed amount for a given service it is called:
    a. accepting assignment
    b. comprehensive insurance
    c. cost shifting
    d. health maintenance

55. C & S tests on patient specimens are performed in:
    a. blood bank
    b. chemistry
    c. immunology
    d. microbiology

56. Electrolyte testing would be performed in:
    a. chemistry
    b. hematology
    c. microbiology
    d. radioimmunoassay

57. Which medical specialty treats patients with blood disorders?
    a. dermatology
    b. hematology
    c. internal medicine
    d. urology

58. Which duty is *not* performed by local public health agencies?
    a. diabetes screening
    b. insect control
    c. licensure of health care personnel
    d. sanitation inspections

59. Blood typing and compatibility testing are performed in:
    a. blood bank
    b. chemistry
    c. coagulation
    d. hematology

60. A sample for fibrin degradation products (FDP) testing would be sent to:
    a. blood bank
    b. chemistry
    c. coagulation
    d. microbiology

61. Which test performed in immunology detects streptococcus infection?
    a. ASO
    b. Monospot
    c. RA
    d. RPR

62. A Pap smear is examined for the presence of cancer cells in this department:
    a. cytology
    b. hematology
    c. histology
    d. microbiology

63. A federal program that provides medical care for the indigent:
    a. homecare services
    b. Medicaid
    c. Medicare
    d. Workers' Compensation

64. Which department performs chemical screening tests on urine specimens?
    a. coagulation
    b. hematology
    c. microbiology
    d. urinalysis

65. Which department would perform an erythrocyte sedimentation rate?
    a. chemistry
    b. hematology
    c. immunology
    d. microbiology

Match the test with the correct department:

66. _____ ABO type
67. _____ antibody screen
68. _____ bilirubin
69. _____ C & S
70. _____ cholesterol
71. _____ glucose
72. _____ HCT
73. _____ K+
74. _____ monospot
75. _____ platelet count
76. _____ PTT
77. _____ retic
78. _____ RPR
79. _____ UA
80. _____ WBC count

    a. blood bank
    b. chemistry
    c. coagulation
    d. hematology
    e. microbiology
    f. serology
    g. urinalysis

Match the organ or body part with the area of medical specialty:

81. _____ brain
82. _____ ear
83. _____ eye
84. _____ heart
85. _____ kidney
86. _____ ovary
87. _____ joint
88. _____ skin
89. _____ stomach
90. _____ thyroid

    a. cardiology
    b. dermatology
    c. endocrinology
    d. gastroenterology
    e. gerontology
    f. gynecology
    g. neurology
    h. ophthalmology
    i. orthopedics
    j. otolaryngology
    k. urology

Match the condition with the medical specialty:

91. _____ anemia
92. _____ arthritis
93. _____ diabetes
94. _____ knee surgery
95. _____ menopause
96. _____ senility
97. _____ skin disorders
98. _____ spinal cord injury
99. _____ tumor
100. _____ urinary tract disease

    a. dermatology
    b. endocrinology
    c. gerontology
    d. gastroenterology
    e. gynecology
    f. hematology
    g. neurology
    h. oncology
    i. orthopedics
    j. rheumatology
    k. urology

ANSWERS TO REVIEW QUESTIONS

1. *b.* The hematology department identifies abnormalities of the blood by analyzing whole blood specimens in automated machines (Fig. 2-1).

2. *a.* The term "outpatient care" is synonymous with "ambulatory care." Ambulatory or outpatient care is offered to those who are able to come to the facility for care and go home the same day. Nonambulatory care is found in tertiary facilities where patients must stay over one or more nights. Nursing home or rehabilitation care is considered nonambulatory for the reasons stated above.

3. *d.* Special chemistry is a subsection of the chemistry department. Some tests performed in this particular section involve the technique called radioimmunoassay which uses radioactively labeled antibodies and antigens to test for minute analytes such as hormones.

4. *c.* Medical Record Technology has recently changed its name to Health Information Technology to more adequately convey its scope of practice. This department maintains patient medical records.

5. *c.* A frozen section is a test performed by a pathologist in the surgical pathology department. Tissue removed during surgery is quickly frozen and a thin slice of the specimen is microscopically examined for abnormalities while the patient is still under anesthesia. Results of the frozen section analysis will determine what further action is taken by the surgeon.

6. *d.* The medical specialty involved in the diagnosis and treatment of joint and muscle disease is called rheumatology.

7. *a.* The chemistry department performs tests to evaluate analytes dissolved

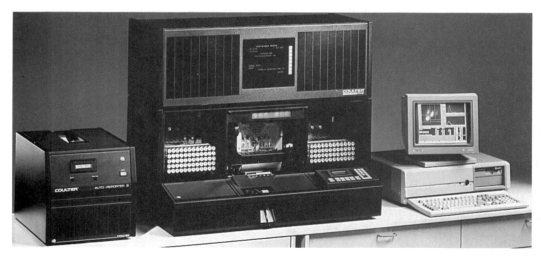

FIGURE 2-1. Coulter STKS System, introduced in 1989, is a fully automated, high-volume hematology analyzer. (Courtesy Coulter Electronics, Inc., Hialeah, FL.)

in the blood plasma. One such analyte is glucose. Glucose levels are evaluated to diagnose or monitor diabetes.

8. *d.* A prothrombin time (protime or PT) is performed in the coagulation department. It is most commonly performed to monitor the effects of coumarin on the coagulation process.

9. *a.* A clinical laboratory scientist (CLS) and a medical technologist (MT) are required to have a bachelor's degree either in medical technology or a chemical or biological science.

10. *c.* The term orthopedic comes from the greek word "orthos" which means "straight" and the root word "pedia" that means child. The term orthopedics is used to describe the medical specialty that treats disorders of the musculoskeletal system.

11. *a.* In some facilities the blood bank department is called "immunohematology."

12. *c.* Inpatient health care facilities (hospitals) are classified in several different ways. One type of classification is based on ownership. Government-owned hospitals include federal facilities such as veterans and Indian health service hospitals, and state facilities such as county and city hospitals. A community hospital is categorized as privately owned and not-for-profit as opposed to a hospital that is owned by investors for profit.

13. *b.* Therapeutic drug monitoring is a team effort and requires cooperation between nursing, pharmacy, and the laboratory for quality results.

14. *c.* The histology department prepares tissue samples for microscopic examination by the pathologist.

15. *c.* Presently, the phlebotomist is not required to have a degree to practice. A few states have a licensure law that includes the phlebotomy personnel. To become nationally certified, a phlebotomist should have a high school degree or GED and have completed a formal, structured program in phlebotomy.

16. *c.* Managed care is the generic term for efficient and cost-effective care and is categorized into three levels: primary, secondary, and tertiary. An appendectomy is more complex than primary care, but routine enough to be done in an outpatient, ambulatory setting, and is classified as secondary care.

17. *c.* The microbiology department places blood specimens in a special media to see if microorganisms might be present in the bloodstream. This process is called blood culture testing.

18. *d.* Sodium and potassium are both electrolytes. They can be ordered as individual tests or together, as part of the electrolyte test.

19. *d.* The position of clinical consultant under CLIA '88 serves as a liaison between the clients and laboratory when reporting and interpreting results.

20. *a.* SMAC (which stands for sequential multiple analyzer that's computerized) is the term for a profile or panel of chemistry tests that evaluate the functioning of several different body systems.

21. *c.* The cytogenetics department performs chromosome studies. Not all laboratories have a cytogenetics department.

22. *b.* As a mechanism for reimbursing professional services, capitation limits payment to providers in an effort to control costs. It is prospective rather than retrospective reimbursement and the amount it is based on is the "going rate." Global capitation means that one fee per month per patient will be paid to providers by the managed care plan.

23. *a.* Health care restructuring has brought managed care to the forefront. Payments to providers who furnish managed care are based on numbers of patients (per capita) serviced rather than the number of services provided (fee for service). This is called capitation payment. Entitlements, such as Medicare and worker's compensations payments, are offered through the government to qualified recipients who have earned these insurance programs through employment. The term "cost shifting" has come about because of the inequities between insurance payments to health providers. For example, a provider may charge more to some payers to cover costs not paid for in entitlement programs.

24. *b.* An HMO charges members a flat fee for a complete package of health care services. The fee is normally paid by the member on a monthly basis and is paid regardless of whether the services are used. An additional fee, called a co-payment, is charged at the time services are used. The amount of the co-payment depends on the type of service rendered.

25. *d.* The respiratory therapy department is responsible for administering oxygen therapy.

26. *b.* The EKG department, often called the Cardiovascular Department, performs diagnostic testing and monitoring of heart patients.

27. *b.* A Coombs test is an antigen-antibody test performed in immunohematology or blood bank. It is used to diagnose various hemolytic anemias.

28. *b.* The CLT and the MLT titles are equivalent. The title depends on the national certification examination they have taken.

29. *d.* ICU designates care of an especially attentive nature given to hospital patients immediately following surgery, accidents, heart attacks, etc. ER medicine is characterized as immediate attention to a patient's traumatic needs or the critically ill, but is intense and short term, unlike ICU.

30. *d.* Public health agencies function at the federal, state, and local level. (See answer to question 58.)

31. *c.* The word "microbiology" means the study of microorganisms. The microbiology department analyzes specimens for the presence of bacteria or microorganisms (Fig. 2-2).

32. *d.* There are three types of care offered in the United States: primary (basic) care through the physician, secondary (more complex therapy) care offered on an outpatient basis, and tertiary care which involves the most complex procedures and sophisticated equipment requiring a stay in an inpatient facility. The term "managed care" refers to efficient, cost-effective methods of

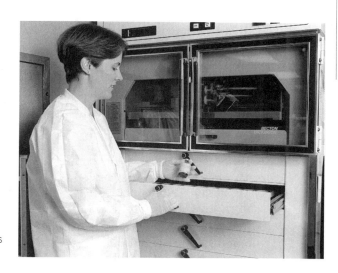

FIGURE 2-2. Microbiologist reviews blood cultures processed by the BACTEC NR-860.

care and applies to all three types of care offered.

33. *c.* The medical specialty that deals with the female reproductive tract and includes prenatal care, labor, and delivery is obstetrics.

34. *d.* The department of radiation therapy uses ionizing radiation in the treatment of malignant tumors.

35. *a.* Toxicology is a subsection of the chemistry department. Tests to determine the presence of poisons or toxic substances in the blood or urine are performed in this area.

36. *d.* A pathologist is a physician who specializes in diagnosing abnormal changes in blood, body fluids, and tissues removed from the body for laboratory analysis.

37. *b.* A CBC is the most common test performed in the hematology department.

38. *b.* Nuclear medicine is a branch of medicine that uses radionuclides to diagnose and treat patients. These radioactive dyes may interfere with certain tests in the laboratory.

39. *a.* CEA is a substance released during malignant tumor growth and is classified as a "tumor marker." It was first associated with cancer of the colon. Because CEA levels increase in other types of cancer as well as some nonmalignant conditions, it is no longer considered specific for colon cancer. Monitoring of CEA levels is, however, considered a useful tool in the treatment and management of certain cancers. CEA levels are performed in the chemistry department.

40. *c.* X-ray procedures and other imaging procedures are functions of the radiology department.

41. *c.* There are two main types of health care facilities: inpatient and outpatient. An inpatient facility is where patients stay overnight. A hospital is primarily an inpatient facility. Outpatient facilities are places where patients receive treatment and go home the same day. Physician's or dentist's offices and day surgery centers are examples of outpatient facilities.

42. *d.* RPR is a common test used in the diagnosis of syphilis. It is performed in the serology department.

43. *b.* Both the MT and the CLS have the same qualification. The title depends on which national certification examination was passed.

44. *b.* Hematology is the department that performs hemograms. A hemogram is a graph of the differential blood count automatically performed when a CBC is ordered.

45. *d.* A routine examination of urine performed in the urinalysis department involves chemical screening tests and a microscopic examination for the presence of blood cells, bacteria, crystals, and other substances.

46. *b.* Physical therapy provides many types of assistance to the patient who has physical handicaps.

47. *b.* EEG performs evoked potential testing to determine muscle function and brain wave mapping to diagnose and monitor neurological disorders (Fig. 2-3).

48. *c.* Managed care was begun for several reasons. Cost-containment for health care was probably the initial reason. More efficient management of patient care while maintaining quality care and keeping costs down is the whole picture.

49. *d.* The new category of acute care personnel is called a PCT. This person is a CNA with additional ancillary skills, but not the nursing skills necessary to qualify as an ADN. An EMT is also a multiskilled person, but one who functions at an emergency level only and is not required to have the nursing skills necessary to qualify for a CNA.

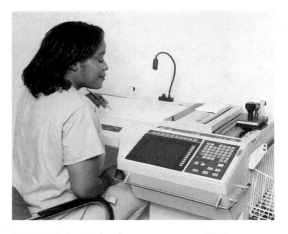

FIGURE 2-3. Technologist monitors an EEG.

50. *b.* The word "onco/logy" when broken down into word root and suffix means *tumor* and *study of*. The term is used to describe the medical specialty that treats patients with tumors.

51. *b.* The CLT is an individual with an associate's degree from a 2-year college or certification from a military or proprietary (private) college.

52. *c.* A subsection of the microbiology department is parasitology where stool specimens are carefully examined in order to identify parasites that are causing infections.

53. *b.* The process used to identify microorganisms and determine the appropriate antibiotic for treatment is called culture and sensitivity (C & S) testing. C & S testing is performed in the microbiology department.

54. *a.* With the advent of DRGs, reimbursement to the provider for services performed was set at a designated amount. If the provider is willing to take exactly what the primary insurer offers as a payment, the provider is said to be accepting what was assigned or "accepting assignment." Cost shifting has come about because of inequities in insurance payments to health providers. For example, a provider may charge more to some payers to cover costs not paid for in entitlement programs. Comprehensive insurance includes both basic and major medical coverage regardless of whether the provider accepts assignment or not.

55. *d.* C & S testing is performed by the microbiology department. Substances suspected of containing pathogenic microorganisms are placed in nutrient media to grow (culture) the microorganism so that it can be identified. Once an organism is identified, an antibiotic susceptibility (sensitivity) test is performed to determine the most effective antibiotic to use for treatment.

56. *a.* The analytes sodium, potassium, and chloride as a group are electrolytes, and testing for these analytes is performed in the chemistry department.

57. *b.* The word root "hem" means blood and "ology" means "study of." Hematology is the medical specialty that treats patients with blood disorders.

58. *c.* Public health agencies take care of large-scale health care problems at the federal, state, and local levels. Their services are designed to be used by the entire population of an area. Licensure of personnel is not part of public health service responsibilities.

59. *a.* Blood bank performs blood typing and compatibility testing.

60. *c.* FDP, also called fibrin split products (FSP), are the end products of the breakdown of fibrin formed during the coagulation process. The test is performed in the coagulation department and is most commonly ordered to diagnose disseminated intravascular coagulation (DIC).

61. *a.* The antistreptolysin O (ASO) titer test is performed to demonstrate the presence of antibodies formed in response to an infection from *Streptococcus* bacteria. A monospot test detects mononucleosis. RA is a rheumatoid arthritis test and rapid plasma reagin (RPR) is a syphilis test.

62. *a.* Cytology is the area in the laboratory in which body fluids and small tissue samples are prepared for examination by a cytologist or pathologist. One of the most common tests performed in this area is the Pap smear.

63. *b.* Medicaid is a state-based federal program that provides medical care for the poor.

64. *d.* Urinalysis is the department in which urine specimens are studied. Part of a complete urinalysis involves performing dipstick chemical screening on each specimen. This chemical screening looks at several dissolved analytes in urine, such as glucose or protein.

65. *b.* The ESR is a whole blood test that is performed in hematology.

66. *a.* blood bank

67. *a.* blood bank

68. *b.* chemistry

69. *e.* microbiology

70. *b.* chemistry

71. *b.* chemistry

72. *d.* hematology

73. *b.* chemistry
74. *f.* serology
75. *d.* hematology
76. *c.* coagulation
77. *d.* hematology
78. *f.* serology
79. *g.* urinalysis
80. *d.* hematology
81. *g.* neurology
82. *j.* otolaryngology
83. *h.* ophthalmology
84. *a.* cardiology
85. *k.* kidney
86. *f.* gynecology

87. *i.* orthopedics
88. *b.* skin
89. *d.* stomach
90. *c.* thyroid
91. *f.* hematology
92. *j.* rheumatology
93. *b.* endocrinology
94. *i.* orthopedics
95. *e.* gynecology
96. *c.* gerontology
97. *a.* dermatology
98. *g.* neurology
99. *h.* oncology
100. *k.* urology

Medical Terminology

REVIEW QUESTIONS

1. What word means "inflammation of the liver"?
   a. cholecystitis
   b. cystosis
   c. hepatitis
   d. microhepatia

2. What does NPO mean?
   a. fasting
   b. newborn
   c. next priority
   d. nothing by mouth

3. What word means "breakdown of glucose"?
   a. antiglycolytic
   b. glycolysis
   c. glycosuria
   d. hemolysis

4. The ability of the body to maintain equilibrium or "steady state" is called:
   a. hematology
   b. homeostasis
   c. hemochromatosis
   d. hemostasis

5. The word root "erythro" means:
   a. cell
   b. earth-like
   c. oxygen
   d. red

6. What word means "hardening of the artery"?
   a. arteriofibrosis
   b. arteriosclerosis
   c. arteriospasm
   d. arteritis

7. What word means "large cell"?
   a. acromegaly
   b. cytoma
   c. macrocyte
   d. microcyte

8. What word means "controlling blood flow"?
   a. anemia
   b. hemostasis
   c. homeostasis
   d. venostasis

9. What word means "condition of clotting"?
   a. hemostasis
   b. thrombosis
   c. vasoconstriction
   d. venostasis

10. Inflammation of a *vein* is:
    a. angitis
    b. cellulitis
    c. phlebitis
    d. vasomyelitis

11. Which of the following terms means muscle pain?
    a. atrophy
    b. myalgia
    c. osteomyelitis
    d. tendinitis

Give the meaning of the following abbreviations using the choices on the right:

Abbreviation	Meaning
12. RBC	a. gynecology
13. RPR	b. lactic dehydrogenase
14. diff	c. phenylketonuria
15. EEG	d. erythrocyte sedimentation rate
16. IM	e. rheumatoid arthritis
17. ASO	f. premature ventricular contraction
18. CMV	g. rapid plasma reagin
19. FUO	h. water reactive
20. DOB	i. weight
21. Rx	j. differential
22. ESR	k. central nervous system
23. W	l. antistreptolysin O
24. LD	m. electroencephalogram
25. O & P	n. nothing by mouth
26. PKU	
27. RA	
28. NPO	o. fever of unknown origin
29. wt	p. intramuscular
	q. electrocardiogram
	r. date of birth
	s. red blood cell count
	t. treatment
	u. ova & parasites
	v. cytomegalovirus

Choose the meaning of the following word roots using the choices on the right:

Word Root	Meaning
30. arteri	a. vessel
31. cardi	b. skin
32. cyte	c. artery
33. derm	d. chest
34. glyc	e. blood
35. hem	f. heart
36. hepat	g. vein
37. onco	h. brain
38. oste	i. liver
39. phleb	j. hard
40. pulmon	k. clot
41. scler	l. cell
42. thromb	m. lung
43. vas	n. bone
	o. tumor
	p. sugar

Choose the meaning of the following prefixes using the choices on the right:

Prefix	Meaning
44. a/an-	a. difficult
45. anti-	b. against
46. brady-	c. unequal
47. dys-	d. without
48. homo-	e. small
49. hypo-	f. low, under
50. micro-	g. large
51. poly-	h. slow
	i. many
	j. same

Choose the meaning of the following suffixes using the choices on the right:

Suffix   **Meaning**

52. -algia   a. tumor
53. -cyte   b. inflammation
54. -emia   c. specialist in the study of
55. -gram   d. deficiency
56. -itis   e. disease
57. -logist   f. condition
58. -lysis   g. cell
59. -oma   h. cutting, incision
60. -osis   i. blood condition
61. -pathy   j. pain
62. -penia   k. bursting forth
63. -rrhage   l. breakdown, destruction
64. -stasis   m. instrument that counts
65. -tomy   n. recording, writing
                     o. enlargement
                     p. stopping, controlling

ANSWERS TO REVIEW QUESTIONS

1. *c.* hepatitis
2. *d.* nothing by mouth
3. *b.* glycolysis
4. *b.* homeostasis
5. *d.* red
6. *a.* arteriosclerosis
7. *c.* macrocyte
8. *b.* hemostasis
9. *b.* thrombosis
10. *c.* phlebitis
11. *b.* myalgia
12. *s.* red blood cell
13. *g.* rapid plasma reagin
14. *j.* differential
15. *m.* electroencephalogram
16. *p.* intramuscular
17. *l.* antistreptolysin O
18. *v.* cytomegalovirus
19. *o.* fever of unknown origin
20. *r.* date of birth
21. *t.* treatment
22. *d.* erythrocyte sedimentation rate
23. *h.* water reactive
24. *b.* lactic dehydrogenase
25. *u.* ova & parasites
26. *c.* phenylketonuria
27. *e.* rheumatoid arthritis
28. *n.* nothing by mouth
29. *i.* weight
30. *c.* artery
31. *f.* heart
32. *l.* cell
33. *b.* skin

34. *p.* sugar
35. *e.* blood
36. *i.* liver
37. *o.* tumor
38. *n.* bone
39. *g.* vein
40. *m.* lung
41. *j.* hard
42. *k.* clot
43. *a.* vessel
44. *d.* without
45. *b.* against
46. *h.* slow
47. *a.* difficult
48. *j.* same
49. *f.* low, under
50. *e.* small
51. *i.* many
52. *j.* pain
53. *g.* cell
54. *i.* blood condition
55. *n.* recording, writing
56. *b.* inflammation
57. *c.* specialist in the study of
58. *l.* breakdown, destruction
59. *a.* tumor
60. *f.* condition
61. *e.* disease
62. *d.* deficiency
63. *k.* bursting forth
64. *p.* stopping, controlling
65. *h.* cutting, incision

Overview of Anatomy and Physiology of the Human Body

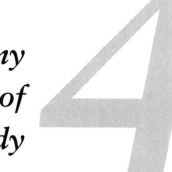

A. **Introduction**
   1. Anatomy
   2. Physiology
B. **Anatomic Position**
   1. Normal
   2. Supine
   3. Prone
C. **Body planes (Includes Diagram)**
   1. Frontal/Coronal
   2. Sagittal/Midsagittal
   3. Transverse
   4. Imaging Procedures
D. **Body Directional Terms**
   1. Anterior (Ventral)/Posterior (Dorsal)
   2. Medial/Lateral
   3. Proximal/Distal
   4. Superior(Cranial)/Inferior(Caudal)
E. **Body Cavities**
   1. Dorsal
      a. Cranial
      b. Spinal
   2. Ventral
      a. Thoracic
      b. Abdominal
      c. Pelvic
F. **Body Functions**
   1. Homeostasis
   2. Metabolism
      a. Catabolism
      b. Anabolism
G. **Body Systems**
   1. Skeletal
      a. Functions
      b. Types of Bones
      c. Disorders
      d. Diagnostic Tests
   2. Muscular
      a. Functions
      b. Types of Muscles
      c. Disorders
      d. Diagnostic Tests
   3. Reproductive
      a. Functions
      b. Structures
      c. Disorders
      d. Diagnostic Tests
   4. Digestive
      a. Functions
      b. Structures
      c. Disorders
      d. Diagnostic Tests
   5. Endocrine
      a. Functions
      b. Glands
      c. Disorders
      d. Diagnostic Tests
   6. Nervous
      a. Functions
      b. Structures
      c. Disorders
      d. Diagnostic Tests
   7. Urinary
      a. Functions
      b. Structures
      c. Disorders
      d. Diagnostic Tests

REVIEW QUESTIONS

1. The gland that releases a hormone that follows diurnal rhythms:
   a. adrenal
   b. pineal
   c. thymus
   d. thyroid

2. Which is *not* a function of the integumentary system?
   a. protection
   b. reception of environmental stimuli
   c. temperature regulation
   d. vitamin C manufacture

3. Which of the following is a test of a digestive system organ?
   a. bilirubin
   b. blood urea nitrogen (BUN)
   c. cortisol
   d. cerebral spinal fluid (CSF) analysis

4. The result of all chemical and physical reactions in the body that are necessary to sustain life is called:
   a. anabolism
   b. cannibalism
   c. catabolism
   d. metabolism

5. Which of the following structures in the skin give rise to fingerprints?
   a. arrector pili
   b. hair follicles
   c. papillae
   d. sebaceous glands

6. The fundamental unit of the nervous system is the:
   a. alveoli
   b. meninges
   c. neuron
   d. pharynx

7. Which body plane divides the body into equal portions?
   a. frontal
   b. midsagittal
   c. sagittal
   d. transverse

8. Which of the following is a nervous system disorder?
   a. hepatitis
   b. multiple sclerosis
   c. nephritis
   d. pruritus

9. An example of a dorsal cavity is the:
   a. abdominal cavity
   b. pelvic cavity
   c. spinal cavity
   d. thoracic cavity

10. Which of the following is a disorder associated with the skeletal system?
   a. atrophy
   b. cholecystitis
   c. multiple sclerosis
   d. osteochondritis

11. A major cause of respiratory distress in infants and young children is:

a. cystic fibrosis
b. emphysema
c. mycobacterium tuberculosis
d. respiratory syncytial virus

12. Simple compounds are transformed by the body into complex compounds by a process called:
a. anabolism
b. catabolism
c. digestion
d. hemoconcentration

13. The ability of oxygen to combine with this substance in the red blood cells increases the amount of oxygen that can be carried in the blood by up to 70 times:
a. carbon dioxide
b. glucose
c. hemoglobin
d. potassium

14. This is the "master gland" of the endocrine system:
a. pineal
b. pituitary
c. thymus
d. thyroid

15. Elimination of waste products is a function of this body system:
a. digestive
b. endocrine
c. nervous
d. skeletal

16. Which of the following is a function of the urinary system? To:
a. maintain electrolyte balance
b. produce heat
c. receive environmental stimuli
d. remove carbon dioxide from the body

17. Which body system produces blood cells?
a. muscular
b. integumentary
c. respiratory
d. skeletal

18. Which of the following is a function of the reproductive system? To produce:

a. gametes
b. hormones
c. sex cells
d. all of the above

19. Female gametes are manufactured in the:
a. cervix
b. fallopian tubes
c. ovaries
d. uterus

20. Which of the following is a test of the urinary system?
a. cholinesterase
b. creatine phosphokinase
c. creatinine clearance
d. pleuracentesis

21. This gland produces "fight or flight" hormones:
a. adrenal
b. pancreas
c. pituitary
d. thyroid

22. Which gland is *not* part of the endocrine system?
a. adrenal
b. pituitary
c. sebaceous
d. thyroid

23. Glomeruli are structures found in which of the following systems:
a. nervous
b. reproductive
c. respiratory
d. urinary

24. The ability of the body to repair and maintain itself to achieve a "steady state" describes what term?
a. anabolism
b. catabolism
c. hemostasis
d. homeostasis

25. Prostate-specific antigen (PSA) is a test of which body system?
a. endocrine
b. nervous

c. reproductive
d. respiratory

26. Infant respiratory distress syndrome in premature infants is most often caused by a lack of:
    a. alveoli
    b. carbon dioxide
    c. hemoglobin
    d. surfactant

27. The gallbladder stores:
    a. bile
    b. hormones
    c. insulin
    d. urine

28. The rapid plasma reagin (RPR) test is a diagnostic test of which of the following body systems?
    a. endocrine
    b. reproductive
    c. respiratory
    d. urinary

29. Which of the following is (are) part of the peripheral nervous system (PNS)?
    a. afferent nerves
    b. brain
    c. CSF
    d. meninges

30. Which gland is most active before birth and during childhood?
    a. adrenal
    b. pituitary
    c. thymus
    d. thyroid

31. Renin is secreted by the:
    a. alveoli
    b. kidneys
    c. ovaries
    d. sudoriferous glands

32. Which of the following types of muscle is under *voluntary* control
    a. cardiac
    b. skeletal
    c. smooth
    d. visceral

33. Which of the following structures is *not* part of the male reproductive system?
    a. epididymis
    b. fallopian tubes
    c. prostate
    d. vas deferens

34. Which of the following body cavities are separated by the diaphragm?
    a. abdominal and thoracic
    b. cranial and spinal
    c. pelvic and abdominal
    d. thoracic and cranial

35. Excessive growth hormone (GH) in adulthood can cause:
    a. acromegaly
    b. Cushing's syndrome
    c. encephalitis
    d. goiter

36. Which of the following is a test of the respiratory system?
    a. arterial blood gases (ABGs)
    b. CSF
    c. thyroid-stimulating hormone (TSH)
    d. urinalysis

37. Which of the following tests is most likely a test of the integumentary system?
    a. ammonia
    b. occult blood
    c. fungal culture
    d. synovial fluid analysis

38. A hormone that increases metabolism is:
    a. cortisol
    b. melatonin
    c. renin
    d. thyroxine

39. The term distal means:
    a. farthest from the point of attachment
    b. higher or above
    c. nearest to the center of the body
    d. toward the back

40. When you are facing someone in normal anatomic position, which body plane are you looking at?
    a. frontal

b. midsagittal
c. sagittal
d. transverse

41. Which of the following structures comprise the central nervous system?
   a. afferent and efferent nerves
   b. brain and spinal cord
   c. sensory and motor nerves
   d. voluntary and involuntary nerves

42. The layer of the skin where mitosis occurs is the:
   a. dermis
   b. germinativum
   c. subcutaneous
   d. none of the above

43. Which of the following is a disorder of the urinary system?
   a. cystitis
   b. renal failure
   c. uremia
   d. all of the above

44. The medical term for elevated blood sugar is:
   a. diabetes
   b. hyperglycemia
   c. hypoglycemia
   d. hypothyroidism

45. Erythropoietin is a hormone secreted by the:
   a. islets of Langerhans
   b. kidneys
   c. pituitary gland
   d. thyroid gland

46. The layer(s) of the skin containing blood vessels is (are):
   a. epidermis only
   b. epidermis and dermis
   c. dermis and subcutaneous
   d. subcutaneous only

47. Functions of the muscular system do *not* include:
   a. stores calcium
   b. produces heat
   c. maintains posture
   d. provides movement

48. Hepatitis is inflammation of the:
   a. gallbladder
   b. kidneys
   c. liver
   d. pancreas

49. What infectious disease affecting the respiratory system is caused by a mycobacterium?
   a. asthma
   b. emphysema
   c. respiratory syncytial virus (RSV)
   d. tuberculosis (TB)

50. Which of the following terms describes the type of cells that make up the epidermis?
   a. epithelial
   b. keratinized
   c. stratified
   d. all of the above

51. T4 & TSH measure the function of which gland?
   a. adrenal
   b. ovaries
   c. pancreas
   d. thyroid

52. The heart and lungs are located in this cavity:
   a. abdominal
   b. cranial
   c. spinal
   d. thoracic

53. GH levels test the functioning of which gland?
   a. adrenal
   b. ovary
   c. parathyroid
   d. pituitary

54. The exchange of O_2 and CO_2 in the lungs takes place in the:
   a. alveoli
   b. bronchi
   c. larynx
   d. trachea

55. Which of the following is a true statement? Your:

a. abdominal cavity is located superior to your diaphragm
b. elbow is on the ventral surface of your arm
c. head is located inferior to your neck
d. little toe is on the lateral surface of your foot

56. Which of the following substances is secreted by the islets of Langerhans of the pancreas?
a. adrenaline
b. estrogen
c. glucose
d. insulin

57. Which of the following structures is part of the digestive system?
a. arrector pili
b. gallbladder
c. seminal vesicle
d. ureter

58. Calcitonin levels test the functioning of which of the following glands?
a. adrenal
b. pituitary
c. thymus
d. thyroid

59. Which of the following laboratory tests is associated with the skeletal system?
a. alkaline phosphatase
b. bilirubin
c. cortisol
d. lactic acid

60. Antidiuretic hormone (ADH) is also called:
a. adrenaline
b. cortisol
c. norepinephrine
d. vasopressin

61. When a person has difficulty breathing, the term used to describe the condition is:
a. asthma
b. dyspnea
c. emphysema
d. pneumonia

62. This body system is responsible for releasing hormones directly into the blood stream:
a. circulatory
b. endocrine
c. respiratory
d. skeletal

63. Which of the following body planes divides the body into upper and lower portions?
a. frontal
b. midsagittal
c. sagittal
d. transverse

64. A disease in which the islets of Langerhans are unable to produce insulin is:
a. diabetes insipidus
b. diabetes mellitus type I
c. diabetes mellitus type II
d. all of the above

65. Which of the following is a nervous system test?
a. BUN
b. CPK
c. CSF analysis
d. glucose

66. Which body system controls and coordinates the activities of all the other body systems?
a. muscular
b. nervous
c. respiratory
d. skeletal

67. Which of the following is a diagnostic test associated with the muscular system?
a. BUN
b. creatine kinase (CK)
c. CSF
d. TSH

68. Which of the following is a disorder of the integumentary system?
a. diabetes
b. impetigo

   c. meningitis
   d. rhinitis

69. The avascular layer of the skin is the:
   a. dermis
   b. epidermis
   c. subcutaneous
   d. none of the above

70. Pancreatitis is a disorder of this system:
   a. digestive
   b. reproductive
   c. respiratory
   d. skeletal

71. Which of the following is a true statement?
   a. a man who is supine is lying down on his stomach
   b. the big toe is on the medial side of the foot
   c. the hand is at the proximal end of the arm
   d. the posterior curvature of the heel is a recommended heel puncture site

72. Which of the following organs has endocrine function?
   a. kidneys
   b. placenta
   c. stomach
   d. all of the above

73. Which of the following are male gametes?
   a. gonads
   b. ovum
   c. spermatozoa
   d. testes

74. Amylase and lipase are diagnostic tests associated with this system:
   a. circulatory
   b. digestive
   c. respiratory
   d. skeletal

75. Wasting or decrease in size of a muscle due to inactivity is called:
   a. atrophy
   b. myalgia
   c. osteomyelitis
   d. tendinitis

ANSWERS TO REVIEW QUESTIONS

1. *b.* The pineal gland secretes the hormone melatonin. Melatonin secretion is inhibited by light and enhanced by darkness. Levels of melatonin in the blood, therefore, follow a diurnal rhythm with levels lowest around noon and highest at night.

2. *d.* Vitamin D, not vitamin C, is manufactured in the skin.

3. *a.* Bilirubin is a liver function test. The liver is an accessory organ of the digestive system. BUN is a kidney function test and therefore a urinary system test. Cortisol is an adrenal function test and therefore an endocrine system test. CSF is a nervous system test.

4. *d.* Metabolism is defined as the sum of all chemical and physical reactions necessary to sustain life. Cannibalism is the eating of human flesh. (See answer to question 12 for anabolism and catabolism.)

5. *c.* Papillae (Fig. 4-1), elevations and depressions in the dermis where it meets the epidermis, form the ridges and grooves of fingerprints.

6. *c.* The neuron is the fundamental unit of the nervous system. The meninges are the covering of the brain and spinal cord. Alveoli and pharynx are structures of the respiratory system.

7. *b.* A midsagittal plane (Fig. 4-2) divides the body into equal right and left portions.

8. *b.* Multiple sclerosis is a disorder involving the myelin sheath of the

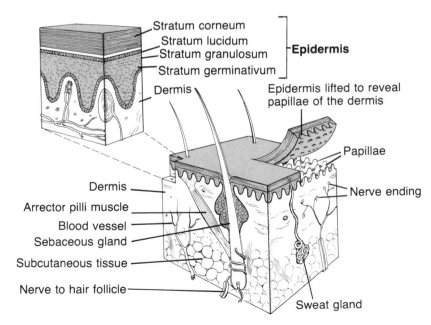

FIGURE 4-1. Cross-section of the skin (Rosdahl C).

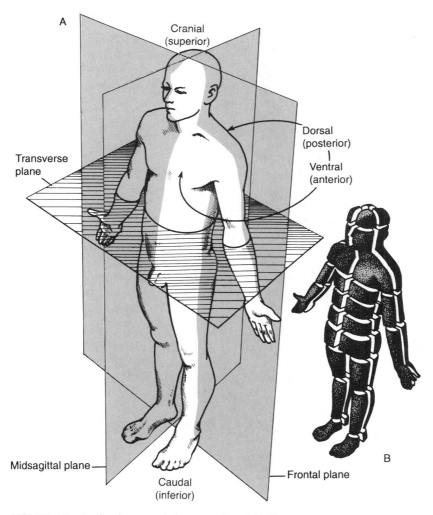

FIGURE 4-2. Body planes and directions (Rosdahl C).

nerves. Hepatitis is liver inflammation. Nephritis is inflammation of the nephrons of the kidneys. Pruritus means itching.

9. *c.* Dorsal refers to the back. Dorsal cavities are to the back of the body. The spinal and cranial cavities are dorsal cavities. The abdominal, pelvic, and thoracic cavities are *ventral* cavities (see Fig. 4-3).

10. *d.* Osteochondritis means inflammation of the bone and cartilage. Atrophy means muscle wasting. Cholecystitis is gallbladder inflammation. Multiple sclerosis is an inflammatory disease of the nervous system that causes degeneration of the myelin sheath of the nerves.

11. *d.* Respiratory syncytial virus causes acute respiratory disease in children.

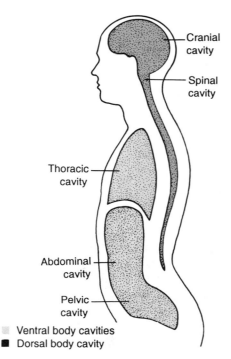

Cranial
cavity

Spinal
cavity

Thoracic
cavity

Abdominal
cavity

Pelvic
cavity

▨ Ventral body cavities
■ Dorsal body cavity

FIGURE 4-3. Side view of body cavities (Rosdahl C).

Cystic fibrosis, emphysema, and mycobacterium tuberculosis can cause respiratory distress in children but are not as common.

12. *a.* Anabolism is the name for the process in which simple compounds are transformed into complex compounds. Catabolism is the process by which complex substances are broken into simple ones. Digestion is the process by which food is broken into simple usable components. Hemoconcentration is a term that means increased large molecules.

13. *c.* The ability of oxygen to combine with a protein in the blood called hemoglobin increases the oxygen-carrying capacity of the blood.

Hemoglobin combined with oxygen is called oxyhemoglobin.

14. *b.* The pituitary gland (Fig. 4-4) releases hormones that stimulate other glands and is therefore referred to as the "master gland."

15. *a.* Elimination of waste products is a function of the digestive system (Fig. 4-5).

16. *a.* The function of the kidneys, which are a part of the urinary system (Fig. 4-6), is to maintain water and electrolyte balance. Electrolytes are sodium, potassium, chloride, and bicarbonate. Heat production is a function of the muscular system. The nervous system and the skin receive environmental stimuli and the circulatory system removes carbon dioxide.

17. *d.* One function of the skeletal system is hematopoiesis or the production of blood cells.

18. *d.* Production of sex cells (gametes) and hormones are functions of the reproductive system.

19. *c.* Female gametes (ova) are manufactured by the ovaries. The uterus is another name for the womb. The fallopian tubes are the pathway through which the ova reach the uterus. The cervix is the neck of the uterus.

20. *c.* Creatinine, a byproduct of muscle energy, is produced at a constant rate and is cleared from the blood by the kidneys. The creatinine clearance test measures the rate that creatinine is cleared from the blood by the kidneys and is a test of kidney function. Creatine phosphokinase is a muscle enzyme and is a test of the muscular system. Cholinesterase is a test that measures the effects of muscle

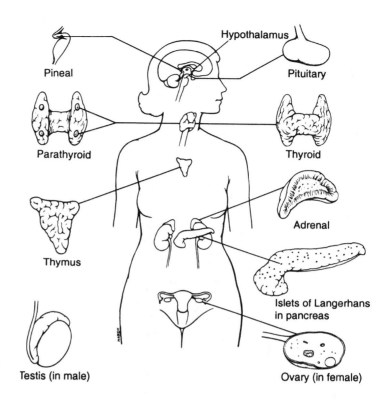

FIGURE 4-4. Glands of the endocrine system (Rosdahl C).

relaxants used in surgery. Pleuracentesis is a surgical puncture of the chest wall to remove fluid.

21. *a.* The adrenal glands (see Fig. 4-4) secrete the hormones epinephrine (adrenaline) and norepinephrine (noradrenaline), also referred to as the "fight or flight" hormones because of their effects when the body is under stress.

22. *c.* Sebaceous glands (see Fig. 4-1) are found in the skin and are part of the integumentary system. They secrete an oily substance called sebum that helps lubricate the skin.

23. *d.* Glomeruli are structures of the kidney which is part of the urinary system.

24. *d.* Homeostasis means "staying the same" and describes the balanced or "steady state" condition that the body strives to maintain. Anabolism is the part of the metabolism process in which the body converts simple substances into complex substances. Catabolism is the process by which the body breaks complex substances into simple ones. Hemostasis is a another term for the coagulation process.

25. *c.* The PSA test is a test associated with the prostate gland which is part of the male reproductive system.

26. *d.* Surfactant is a fluid substance that coats the thin walls of the alveoli and keeps them from collapsing. Premature infants often lack sufficient surfactant to keep their lungs from collapsing.

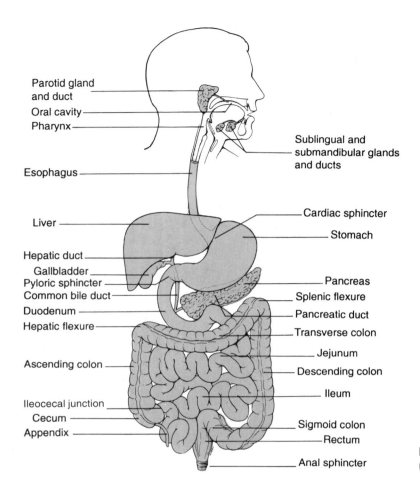

Parotid gland and duct

Oral cavity

Pharynx

Esophagus

Liver

Hepatic duct

Gallbladder

Pyloric sphincter

Common bile duct

Duodenum

Hepatic flexure

Ascending colon

Ileocecal junction

Cecum

Appendix

Sublingual and submandibular glands and ducts

Cardiac sphincter

Stomach

Pancreas

Splenic flexure

Pancreatic duct

Transverse colon

Jejunum

Descending colon

Ileum

Sigmoid colon

Rectum

Anal sphincter

FIGURE 4-5. The digestive system (Rosdahl C).

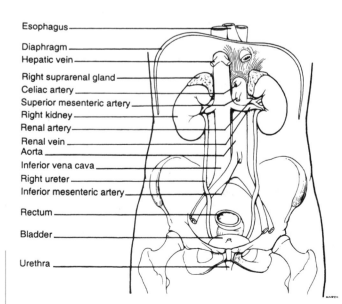

Esophagus

Diaphragm

Hepatic vein

Right suprarenal gland

Celiac artery

Superior mesenteric artery

Right kidney

Renal artery

Renal vein

Aorta

Inferior vena cava

Right ureter

Inferior mesenteric artery

Rectum

Bladder

Urethra

FIGURE 4-6. The urinary system (Rosdahl C).

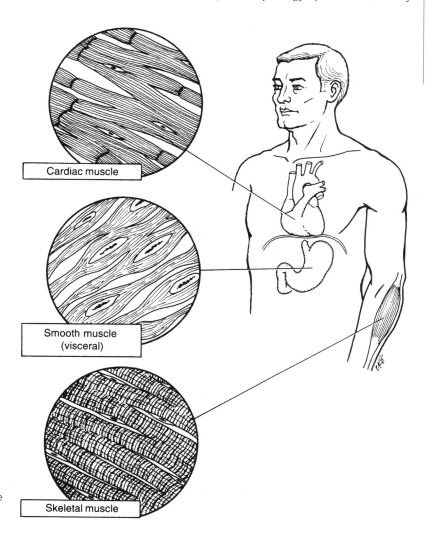

FIGURE 4-7. Types of muscle tissue.

Cardiac muscle

Smooth muscle (visceral)

Skeletal muscle

27. *a.* The gallbladder (see Fig. 4-5) serves as a storage pouch for bile.

28. *b.* The RPR test is a test for syphilis which is a sexually transmitted disease of the reproductive system.

29. *a.* Afferent nerves are part of the PNS (see answer to question 41). The brain and spinal fluid and meninges are part of the central nervous system.

30. *c.* The thymus gland (see Fig. 4-4), located in the chest behind the sternum, functions in the development of immunity and is most active before birth and during childhood.

31. *b.* Renin, a hormone secreted by the kidneys, increases blood pressure.

32. *b.* Skeletal muscle is under voluntary control. Cardiac and visceral (smooth) muscle are under involuntary control (Fig. 4-7).

33. *b.* The epididymis, prostate, and vas deferens are structures of the male

reproductive system. The fallopian tubes are structures of the female reproductive system (Fig. 4-8).

34. *a.* The diaphragm is a muscular structure separating the thoracic cavity from the abdominal cavity.

35. *a.* Acromegaly is a condition characterized by the overgrowth of bones in the hands, feet, and face caused by excessive growth hormone in adulthood. Cushing's syndrome is caused by an excess of cortisone.

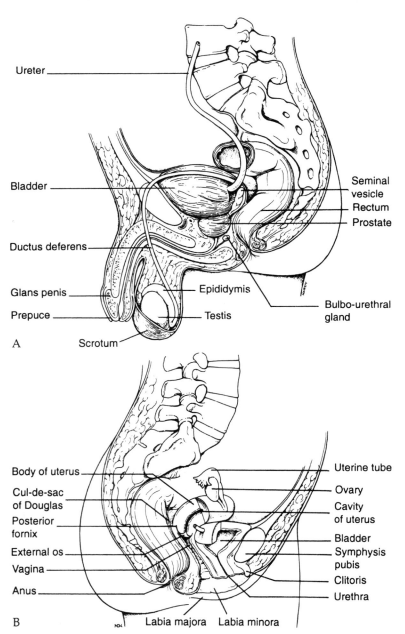

FIGURE 4-8. **(A)** Male reproductive system; **(B)** Female reproductive system (Rosdahl C).

Goiter is a term for an enlargement of the thyroid gland. Encephalitis means inflammation of the brain.

36. *a.* ABGs assess a patient's oxygenation and ventilation status which are functions of the respiratory system. CSF is a nervous system test. TSH is a pituitary hormone that stimulates the thyroid and is a thyroid function test. A urinalysis is a urinary system test.

37. *c.* Fungal cultures are often performed on skin scrapings. The skin is part of the integumentary system. Ammonia, a liver function test, and occult blood, a test for hidden blood in feces, are digestive system tests. Synovial fluid comes from joint cavities, part of the skeletal system.

38. *d.* Thyroxine is a hormone released by the thyroid (see Fig. 4-4) that increases the metabolic rate.

39. *a.* Distal means farthest from the center of the body, origin, or point of attachment. Superior means higher or above. Proximal means nearest to the center of the body. Dorsal refers to the back.

40. *a.* The frontal plane divides the body vertically into front and back portions. When you are facing someone in anatomic position, he or she is also facing you which means you are seeing the frontal plane. A sagittal plane divides the body into right and left portions. A midsagittal plane divides a body into equal right and left portions. A transverse plane divides the body into upper and lower portions (see Fig. 4-2).

41. *b.* The central nervous system (Fig. 4-9) is composed of the brain and spinal cord. The afferent and efferent nerves, sensory and motor nerves, and voluntary and involuntary nerves are all part of the PNS.

42. *b.* The only layer of the skin where mitosis (cell division) occurs is a layer called the stratum germinativum.

43. *d.* Cystitis is inflammation of the bladder. Renal failure means kidney failure. Uremia is a build up of waste products in the body caused by impaired kidney function.

44. *b.* Hyperglycemia is the term for abnormally increased blood sugar. Hypoglycemia is a term for abnormally decreased blood sugar. Diabetes is a general term for diseases characterized by abnormally increased urination. Hypothyroidism is a disease caused by decreased thyroid secretion.

45. *b.* The kidneys release erythropoietin, a hormone that stimulates red blood cell production.

46. *c.* Blood vessels are found in the dermis and subcutaneous layers of the skin. The epidermis is avascular, which means it does not contain blood vessels.

47. *a.* Calcium storage is a function of the skeletal system.

48. *c.* Hepatitis comes from the greek word "hepatos" meaning liver. The suffix "itis" means inflammation. The term for inflammation of the gallbladder is *cholecystitis*. Kidney inflammation is called *nephritis*. Inflammation of the pancreas is called *pancreatitis*.

49. *d.* TB is caused by *Mycobacterium tuberculosis*. This disease once considered rare in the United States is now in resurgence because of antibiotic resistance of the organism and the increase of world travel. RSV is caused by, as the name implies, a virus, not a mycobacterium. Asthma

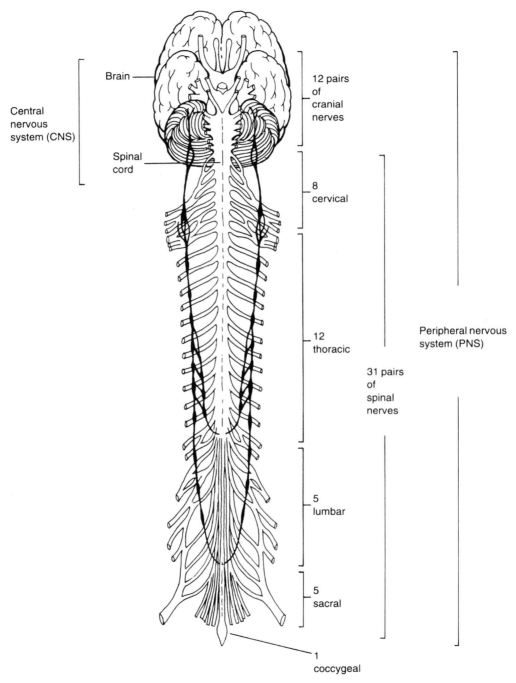

FIGURE 4-9. The nervous system.

and emphysema are conditions related to difficulty in breathing and are not infectious diseases.

50. *d.* Some cells of the epidermis can be described as stratified (layered), keratinized (hardened), epithelial cells.

51. *d.* Thyroxine (T4), a hormone released by the thyroid gland (see Fig. 4-6), increases metabolic rate. TSH is released by the pituitary to stimulate the thyroid. Both T4 and TSH are common tests of thyroid function.

52. *d.* The heart and lungs are located in the thoracic or chest cavity. (See Fig. 4-2.)

53. *d.* GH is secreted by the pituitary gland.

54. *a.* The larynx, trachea, bronchi, and alveoli are all parts of the respiratory system (Fig. 4-10), but the exchange of oxygen and carbon dioxide occurs in the alveoli.

55. *d.* The little toe is on the outer or lateral side of the foot. The abdominal cavity is inferior or below the diaphragm. The elbow is on the back or dorsal surface of the arm. The head is above or superior to the neck.

56. *d.* The islets of Langerhans are part of the endocrine system. They secrete insulin which is necessary for the cells to be able to utilize glucose. Adrenaline is secreted by the adrenal glands. Estrogen is secreted by the ovaries in the female reproductive system.

57. *b.* The gallbladder (see Fig. 4-5) is an accessory organ of the digestive system. Arrector pili are structures in the skin. Seminal vesicles are part of the male reproductive system. Ureters are structures of the urinary system.

58. *d.* Calcitonin is a hormone secreted by the thyroid that regulates the amount of calcium in the blood.

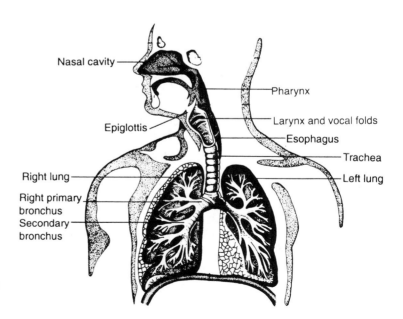

FIGURE 4-10. The respiratory system (Rosdahl C).

59. *a.* Alkaline phosphatase is an enzyme that functions in the mineralization process of bone. Bilirubin is a liver function test. Cortisol is an endocrine system test. Lactic acid is a test associated with the muscular system.

60. *d.* Vasopressin is another name for ADH, which is secreted by the pituitary and decreases urine production.

61. *b.* The prefix "dys-" means difficult. "Pnea" comes from "pnoe" which means breathing. Asthma is a condition characterized by difficult breathing (dyspnea) accompanied by wheezing. Emphysema is a chronic obstructive pulmonary disease. Pneumonia is inflammation of the lungs most commonly caused by bacteria, viruses, or chemical irritation.

62. *b.* The endocrine system releases hormones directly into the blood stream.

63. *d.* The transverse plane divides the body into upper and lower portions (see Fig. 4-2).

64. *b.* In diabetes mellitus type I, also called insulin-dependent diabetes, the body is totally unable to produce insulin. In diabetes mellitus type II, also called noninsulin-dependent diabetes, the body is able to produce insulin, but either the amount produced is not sufficient or the insulin is not being properly used by the body. In diabetes insipidus, a condition characterized by increased thirst and increased urine production, is caused by inadequate secretion of antidiuretic hormone.

65. *c.* CSF is a clear, plasma-like fluid that fills the space between the meninges and the spinal cord and brain. BUN is a measure of the nitrogen portion of urine and is a kidney function test. Creatine phosphokinase (CPK) is a muscle enzyme. Glucose is a product of carbohydrate metabolism and a test of the digestive system.

66. *b.* The nervous system controls and coordinates the activities of all body systems. It does this by means of electrical impulses and chemical substances sent to and received from all parts of the body.

67. *b.* CK is an enzyme present in skeletal and heart muscle. BUN is a urinary system test. CSF is a nervous system test. TSH is an endocrine system test.

68. *b.* The skin is part of the integumentary system. Impetigo is an inflammatory condition of the skin most often caused by staphylococcus or streptococcus infection. It is characterized by isolated blisters that rupture and crust over.

69. *b.* Avascular means "without blood vessels." The epidermis of the skin does not contain blood vessels. The blood vessels are in the dermis and subcutaneous layers of the skin.

70. *a.* Pancreatitis means inflammation of the pancreas. The pancreas is an accessory organ of the digestive system.

71. *b.* Medial means toward the midline of the body. The big toe is on the inner side of the foot which is the side closest to the midline of the body. A man who is in a supine position is lying down on his back. The hand is at the distal end of the arm. The posterior curvature of the heel is *not* a recommended site for heel puncture.

72. *d.* The kidneys manufacture the hormones renin and erythropoietin,

the placenta produces chorionic gonadotropin, and the stomach secretes gastrin.

73. **c.** Male gametes or sex cells are called spermatozoa. An ovum is a female gamete. Gonads are the glands that manufacture the gametes. The male gonads are the testes.

74. **b.** Amylase and lipase are enzymes produced by the pancreas (an accessory organ of the digestive system) that aid the digestive process.

75. **a.** Atrophy means muscle wasting. Myalgia means muscle pain. Osteomyelitis means bone inflammation. Tendinitis means tendon inflammation.

The Circulatory System

A. **The Heart**
   1. Structures
      a. Layers
      b. Chambers
      c. Valves
      d. Coronary Arteries
      e. Other Structures
   2. Functions
      a. Cardiac Cycle
         (1) Systole/Diastole
         (2) Electrical System
         (3) Electrocardiogram
      b. Heart Beat
      c. Heart Rate
      d. Pulse
      e. Blood Pressure
   3. Disorders
   4. Diagnostic Tests
B. **The Vascular System**
   1. Functions
      a. Pulmonary Circulation
      b. Systemic Circulation
   2. Blood Vessels
      a. Types
         (1) Arteries
         (2) Veins
         (3) Capillaries
      b. Structure
         (1) Layers
         (2) Valves
      c. Functions
   3. Flow of Blood
   4. Related Anatomy of the Arm and Leg
      a. Antecubital Fossa
      b. Antecubital Veins Subject to Venipuncture
      c. Other Arm and Hand Veins
      d. Leg, Ankle, and Foot Veins
      e. Arteries Subject to Puncture
      f. Median Cutaneous Nerve
   5. Disorders
   6. Diagnostic Tests
C. **The Blood**
   1. Composition
      a. Plasma
      b. Formed Elements
         (1) Types
         (2) Description
         (3) Function
         (4) Lifespan
   2. Blood Type
      a. Antigens/Antibodies
      b. Transfusion Reaction
      c. The ABO Blood Group System
      d. The Rh System
         (1) Sensitization
         (2) Hemolytic Disease of the Newborn
         (3) Rh Immunoglobulin
         (4) Crossmatch
   3. Types of Blood Specimens
      a. Serum
      b. Plasma
      c. Whole Blood
   4. Disorders of the Blood
   5. Diagnostic Tests
D. **Hemostasis**
   1. Coagulation Process
      a. Primary/Secondary Hemostasis
      b. Stages
         (1) Vasoconstriction
         (2) Platelet Plug Formation
         (3) Fibrin Clot Formation
         (4) Fibrinolysis

REVIEW QUESTIONS

Using the choices on the right, identify the structures of the heart indicated by the arrows in Figure 5-1:

1. _____
2. _____
3. _____
4. _____
5. _____
6. _____
7. _____
8. _____

   a. aorta
   b. right atrium
   c. left atrium
   d. right ventricle
   e. left ventricle
   f. bicuspid valve
   g. tricuspid valve
   h. pulmonic valve
   i. aortic valve
   j. superior vena cava
   k. inferior vena cava
   l. right pulmonary artery
   m. left pulmonary artery
   n. right pulmonary vein
   o. left pulmonary vein

9. The middle layer of heart muscle is called the:
   a. endocardium
   b. epicardium
   c. myocardium
   d. pericardium

10. The function of the left ventricle is to deliver:
   a. deoxygenated blood into the pulmonary artery
   b. oxygenated blood into the aorta
   c. oxygenated blood into the pulmonary vein
   d. oxygenated blood to the left atrium

11. How many chambers does the human heart have?
   a. 1
   b. 2
   c. 3
   d. 4

12. The medical term for a heart attack is:
   a. arrhythmia
   b. ischemia
   c. myocardial infarction
   d. tachycardia

13. The receiving chambers of the heart are the:
   a. atria
   b. chordae tendineae
   c. vena cavae
   d. ventricles

14. The heart is surrounded by a thin, fluid-filled sac called the:
   a. endocardium
   b. epicardium
   c. myocardium
   d. pericardium

15. The lower chambers of the heart are called:
   a. atria
   b. septum
   c. valves
   d. ventricles

16. On an electrocardiogram (ECG) tracing, which wave represents the activity of the ventricles?

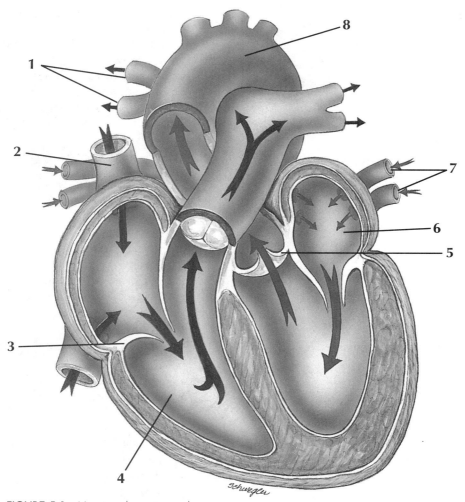

FIGURE 5-1. Heart and great vessels.

a. P and T
b. P only
c. QRS and P
d. QRS and T

17. The structure dividing the right and left halves of the heart is called:
a. atrium
b. chordae tendineae
c. pericardium
d. septum

18. The heart receives blood to supply its own needs via the:

a. coronary arteries
b. pulmonary arteries
c. vena cavae
d. venules

19. The relaxing phase of the cardiac cycle is called:
a. bradycardia
b. diastole
c. infarction
d. systole

20. The heart's "pacemaker" is the:

a. atrioventricular node
b. bundle of His
c. semilunar valve
d. sinoatrial node

21. A cardiac cycle lasts approximately:
    a. 0.5 seconds
    b. 0.8 seconds
    c. 1.5 seconds
    d. 8 seconds

22. Electrical impulses of the heart can be monitored by this test.
    a. ABGs
    b. CK
    c. EEG
    d. ECG

23. On an ECG tracing, atrial activity is represented by the:
    a. P wave
    b. QRS complex
    c. T wave
    d. none of the above

24. The right atrioventricular valve is also called the:
    a. bicuspid valve
    b. mitral valve
    c. pulmonary valve
    d. tricuspid valve

25. Abnormal heart sounds are called:
    a. arrhythmia
    b. extrasystoles
    c. fibrillations
    d. murmurs

26. Blood vessels that carry blood away from the heart are called:
    a. arteries
    b. capillaries
    c. veins
    d. vena cavae

27. A person's pulse is created by a wave of pressure caused by:
    a. atrial contraction
    b. atrial relaxation
    c. ventricular contraction
    d. ventricular relaxation

28. What keeps the blood moving through the venous system?

a. expansion and contraction of the arteries
b. movement of fluid through the lymph system veins
c. pressure from the heart contractions
d. skeletal muscle movement and the opening and closing of valves within the veins

29. An abnormally fast heart rate is called:
    a. bradycardia
    b. extrasystole
    c. fibrillation
    d. tachycardia

30. Which of the following is a normal blood pressure reading:
    a. 60/40
    b. 80/120
    c. 100/120
    d. 120/80

31. An infection of the lining of the heart is called:
    a. angina pectoris
    b. aortic stenosis
    c. endocarditis
    d. pericarditis

32. Which of the following are cardiac enzyme tests?
    a. alkaline phosphatase, SGPT
    b. BUN, PT
    c. CPK, LDH
    d. GTT, ESR

33. Systolic pressure measures pressure in the arteries during:
    a. atrial contraction
    b. ventricular contraction
    c. ventricular relaxation
    d. none of the above

34. The pulmonary circulation:
    a. carries deoxygenated blood to the lungs and returns oxygenated blood to the heart
    b. carries oxygenated blood from the heart to the tissues

c. delivers blood from the heart to the aorta

d. returns deoxygenated blood to the heart

35. Normal systemic arterial blood is:
    a. blue
    b. bright cherry red
    c. dark bluish red
    d. reddish blue

36. The largest artery in the body is the:
    a. aorta
    b. carotid
    c. femoral
    d. vena cava

37. The pulmonary vein carries:
    a. arterial blood
    b. lymph fluid
    c. oxygen-rich blood
    d. oxygen-poor blood

38. A sphygmomanometer is a/an:
    a. blood pressure cuff
    b. electrocardiogram
    c. machine that records brain waves
    d. pacemaker

39. The smallest branches of veins are called:
    a. arterioles
    b. capillaries
    c. lumen
    d. venules

40. Which blood vessel is not part of the systemic circulation?
    a. brachial artery
    b. cephalic vein
    c. pulmonary artery
    d. vena cava

41. The longest vein in the body is the:
    a. aorta
    b. femoral
    c. saphenous
    d. vena cava

42. Tiny one-cell-thick blood vessels are called:
    a. arterioles
    b. capillaries
    c. vena cavae
    d. venules

43. Which of the following blood vessels carries oxygenated blood?
    a. brachial vein
    b. pulmonary vein
    c. pulmonary artery
    d. superior vena cava

44. The outer layer of a blood vessel is called the tunica:
    a. adventitia
    c. interna
    d. intima
    d. media

45. The internal space of a blood vessel is called the:
    a. endothelium
    b. lumen
    c. intima
    d. tunica media

46. The layers of arteries differ from the layers of veins in that the:
    a. inner lining is thicker in veins
    b. outer layer of arteries is thinner
    c. muscle layer of veins is more elastic
    d. muscle layer is thicker in arteries

47. The structure in Figure 5-2 is a/an:
    a. artery
    b. capillary

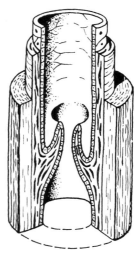

FIGURE 5-2. Blood vessel cross section.

c. vein
d. none of the above

48. Which of the following represents the proper direction that the blood flows?
    a. arteries, veins, capillaries
    b. arterioles, capillaries, venules
    c. capillaries, arterioles, arteries
    d. veins, venules, capillaries

49. The inner layer of a blood vessel is called the:
    a. lumen
    b. tunica adventitia
    c. tunica intima
    d. tunica media

50. The left ventricle delivers blood to the:
    a. aorta
    b. left atrium
    c. pulmonary artery
    d. pulmonary vein

51. Which is the proper order of vein selection for venipuncture?
    a. basilic, cephalic, median cubital
    b. cephalic, median cubital, basilic
    c. median cubital, basilic, cephalic
    d. median cubital, cephalic, basilic

52. Oxygen and nutrients diffuse through the walls of the:
    a. alveoli
    b. arterioles
    c. capillaries
    d. venules

53. The antecubital fossa is located:
    a. anterior to and distal to the elbow
    c. anterior to and distal to the ankle
    b. posterior to and proximal to the elbow
    d. proximal to the wrist

54. A blood clot circulating in the bloodstream is called a/an:
    a. aneurism
    b. embolism
    c. embolus
    d. thrombus

Identify the veins in Figure 5-3 using the choices to the right:

55. _____   a. basilic
56. _____   b. brachial
57. _____   c. cephalic
              d. median cubital
              e. radial

58. The basilic vein is the third choice for venipuncture because it is:
    a. more painful when punctured
    b. near a major nerve
    c. near the brachial artery
    d. all of the above

59. A phlebotomist is allowed to perform a venipuncture on an ankle vein when:
    a. the patient has intravenous catheters in both arms
    b. the patient's physician has given permission to do so
    c. there are no acceptable antecubital or hand veins
    d. there are no other accessible veins and the patient has no coagulation problems

60. Which of the following are a normal part of the plasma portion of the blood?
    a. antibodies
    b. bacteria
    c. platelets
    d. red blood cells

61. What is the medical term for vein inflammation?
    a. embolism
    b. hemostasis
    c. phlebitis
    d. thrombosis

62. Which of the following is a vascular system test?
    a. bilirubin
    b. CSF
    c. DIC
    d. glucose

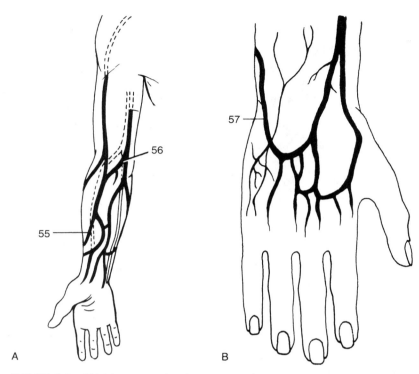

FIGURE 5-3. **(A)** Major superficial arm veins subject to venipuncture; **(B)** Hand veins subject to venipuncture (Timby BK, Lewis LW).

63. Lipid accumulation on the intima of an artery is called:
    a. atherosclerosis
    b. cholesterol
    c. endocarditis
    d. phlebitis

64. A localized dilation or bulging of an artery is called:
    a. an aneurism
    b. an embolism
    c. arteriosclerosis
    d. thrombophlebitis

65. Inflammation of a vein in conjunction with formation of a blood clot is called:
    a. phlebitis
    b. sclerosis
    c. thrombophlebitis
    d. vasculitis

66. Normal adult blood volume is approximately:
    a. 2 L
    b. 4 L
    c. 5 L
    d. 8 L

67. The normal composition of blood is approximately:
    a. 10% plasma; 90% formed elements
    b. 30% plasma; 70% formed elements
    c. 55% plasma; 45% formed elements
    d. 90% plasma; 10% formed elements

68. Normal plasma is a:
    a. clear, colorless fluid that is 10% solutes
    b. clear, pale yellow fluid that is 90% water

c. cloudy, colorless fluid that is 45% solutes

d. hazy, pale yellow fluid that is 55% water

69. When the hand is in pronation the cephalic vein is located in line with the:
    a. femoral artery
    b. radial artery
    c. little finger
    d. thumb

70. Which cell is the most numerous cell in the blood?
    a. platelet
    b. red blood cell
    c. reticulocyte
    d. white blood cell

71. Which blood cell contains a nucleus?
    a. erythrocyte
    b. leukocyte
    c. thrombocyte
    d. reticulocyte

72. A reticulocyte count measures immature:
    a. platelets
    b. neutrophils
    c. red blood cells
    d. white blood cells

73. Which blood cell increases in allergic reactions and pinworm infestations?
    a. eosinophil
    b. monocyte
    c. red blood cell
    d. segmented neutrophil

74. How large is a normal erythrocyte?
    a. 4–5 µm
    b. 7–8 µm
    c. 8–10 µm
    d. 10–12 µm

75. Where are leukocytes produced?
    a. blood stream
    b. bone marrow
    c. kidneys
    d. liver

76. What is the primary function of red blood cells?
    a. deliver nutrients to the cells of the body
    b. produce antibodies
    c. transport carbon dioxide from the tissues to the lungs
    d. transport oxygen from the lungs to the tissues

77. A leukocyte is a:
    a. lymph node
    b. platelet
    c. red blood cell
    d. white blood cell

78. Which blood cell has the ability to pass through the blood vessel walls?
    a. erythrocyte
    b. leukocyte
    c. reticulocyte
    d. thrombocyte

79. Which type of cell destroys pathogens by phagocytosis?
    a. erythrocyte
    b. neutrophil
    c. red blood cell
    d. thrombocyte

80. Which of the following is a another term for neutrophils?
    a. eos
    b. basos
    c. monos
    d. polys

81. Which formed element is first on the scene when an injury occurs?
    a. platelet
    b. red blood cell
    c. reticulocyte
    d. white blood cell

82. Which of the following is described as an anuclear, biconcave disc?
    a. erythrocyte
    b. granulocyte
    c. leukocyte
    d. thrombocyte

83. Which type of cell is sometimes called a macrophage?
    a. eosinophil
    b. basophil
    c. lymphocyte
    d. monocyte

84. Which type of cells give rise to plasma cells that produce antibodies?
    a. eosinophils
    b. lymphocytes
    c. monocytes
    d. neutrophils

85. Neutrophils are sometimes called segs because they have segmented:
    a. cytoplasm
    b. granules
    c. nuclei
    d. none of the above

86. Platelets are also called:
    a. erythrocytes
    b. leukocytes
    c. segs
    d. thrombocytes

87. A platelet is actually a part of a cell called a:
    a. granulocyte
    b. macrophage
    c. megakaryocyte
    d. T-lymphocyte

88. An individual's blood type is determined by the presence or absence of a certain type of:
    a. antibody present on the white blood cells
    b. antibody present on the red blood cells
    c. antigen present on the white blood cells
    d. antigen present on the red blood cells

89. To prevent sensitization, Rh immunoglobulin is given to a/an:
    a. pregnant woman if there is bleeding during the pregnancy
    b. Rh-negative mother on delivery of an Rh-positive baby
    c. Rh-positive baby immediately after birth
    d. Rh-positive mother on delivery of an Rh-negative baby

90. A person who becomes "sensitized" to the Rh factor:
    a. has the Rh antigen
    b. is Rh positive
    c. may produce antibodies to the Rh factor
    d. should not have children

91. A person who has A negative blood has red blood cells that:
    a. have the A antigen and lack the Rh antigen
    b. have the A antigen and the Rh antigen
    c. lack the A antigen and have the Rh antigen
    d. lack the A antigen and the Rh antigen

92. Severe hemolytic disease of the newborn is most often caused by:
    a. ABO incompatibility between mother and baby
    b. an incompatible blood transfusion
    c. preformed Rh antibodies present shortly after birth
    d. sensitization of an Rh-negative mother from a previous Rh-positive baby

93. Whole blood is made up of:
    a. aggregated platelets and water
    b. formed elements suspended in plasma
    c. serum and cells
    d. serum and clotted red blood cells

94. The liquid portion of a clotted specimen is called:
    a. fibrinogen
    b. plasma
    c. saline
    d. serum

95. The clear liquid portion of an anticoagulated specimen that has been centrifuged is called:

a. buffy coat
b. plasma
c. saline
d. serum

96. Figure 5-4 shows a centrifuged plasma specimen. Identify the portion of the specimen indicated by the arrow.
    a. buffy coat
    b. plasma
    c. serum
    d. red blood cells

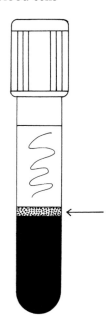

FIGURE 5-4. Centrifuged plasma specimen.

97. How can you visually tell serum from plasma?
    a. serum is clear, plasma is cloudy
    b. serum is fluid, plasma is a gel
    c. serum is pale yellow, plasma is colorless
    d. you cannot visually tell serum from plasma

98. How soon should a blood smear be made from an ethylenediaminetetraacetate (EDTA) specimen? Within:

a. 5 minutes
b. 30 minutes
c. 60 minutes
d. 12 hours

99. The most common anticoagulants prevent clotting by:
    a. enhancing thrombin formation and releasing calcium
    b. inhibiting glucose or binding fibrinogen
    c. inhibiting thrombin or binding calcium
    d. removing fibrinogen

100. It is preferable to perform "stat" chemistry tests on plasma rather than serum because plasma:
    a. is more stable than serum
    b. is ready for testing sooner than serum.
    c. results are more accurate
    d. tests require a smaller volume of specimen

101. A test that assesses platelet plug formation:
    a. bleeding time (BT)
    b. fibrin degradation products (FDP)
    c. prothrombin time (PT)
    d. partial thromboplastin time (PTT)

102. Which of the following statements is *not* true? Serum:
    a. is collected without an anticoagulant
    b. contains fibrinogen
    c. is normally clear, pale yellow in color
    d. is suitable for most chemistry determinations

103. A person with thrombocytosis has:
    a. abnormally decreased platelets
    b. abnormally functioning platelets
    c. abnormally increased platelets
    d. normal platelets

104. A disease characterized by an abnormally decreased red blood cell count:
    a. anemia
    b. leukopenia

c. polycythemia
d. thrombocytopenia

105. The process of coagulation is also called:
    a. hemoconcentration
    b. hemolysis
    c. hemostasis
    d. homeostasis

106. Which of the following is a test of the formed elements?
    a. BUN
    b. CBC
    c. electrolytes
    d. glucose

107. Hemostasis refers to:
    a. broken red blood cells
    b. increased large molecules in the bloodstream
    c. keeping the body in equilibrium
    d. the coagulation process

108. An abnormal increase in white blood cells is called:
    a. leukemia
    b. leukocytosis
    c. leukopenia
    d. leukopoiesis

109. The ion required in the coagulation process where prothrombin is converted to thrombin is:
    a. calcium
    b. chloride
    c. potassium
    d. sodium

110. The extrinsic pathway of coagulation is initiated by:
    a. events within the bloodstream
    b. factor VIII
    c. platelet plug formation
    d. tissue injury

111. The first stage in the hemostatic process is:
    a. fibrin clot formation
    b. fibrinolysis
    c. platelet plug formation
    d. vasoconstriction

112. Which test is *not* used to diagnose blood disorders?
    a. complete blood count
    b. creatinine
    c. ferritin
    d. hemoglobin

113. Which stages of the coagulation process are called *primary hemostasis*?
    a. fibrin clot formation and fibrinolysis
    b. fibrin clot formation only
    c. platelet plug formation and fibrin clot formation
    d. vasoconstriction and platelet plug formation

114. Lymph fluid is most like:
    a. serum
    b. plasma
    c. urine
    d. whole blood

115. A disease caused most often by the lack of factor VIII:
    a. disseminated intravascular coagulation
    b. hemophilia
    c. leukemia
    d. thrombocytopenia

116. Coagulation problems may result from liver disease because the liver:
    a. filters blood improperly when diseased
    b. manufactures coagulation factors
    c. releases calcium
    d. removes red blood cells

117. Which stage of the coagulation process involves the action of the enzyme plasmin?
    a. fibrin clot formation
    b. fibrinolysis
    c. platelet plug formation
    d. vasoconstriction

118. Tests that measure the functioning of primary hemostasis:
    a. fibrin degradation products and bleeding time
    b. platelet count and bleeding time

c. platelet count and protime
d. protime and partial thromboplastin time

119. Obstruction of a blood vessel by an embolus causes:
a. a thrombus
b. an embolism
c. atherosclerosis
d. thrombophlebitis

120. Which of the following is a coagulation test?
a. electrolytes
b. glycohemoglobin
c. hemoglobin
d. protime

121. When the arm is in the anatomic position, the basilic vein is:
a. in line with the middle finger
b. in the center of the antecubital fossa
c. on the same side as the little finger
d. on the same side as the thumb

122. Lymph fluid originates from:
a. excess tissue fluid
b. lymph nodes
c. the liver
d. the kidneys

123. A venipuncture site is normally healed by:
a. fibrin clot formation
b. fibrinolysis
c. platelet plug formation
d. vasoconstriction only

124. A malignant lymphoid tumor:
a. lymphadenopathy
b. lymphangitis
c. lymphoma
d. lymphosarcoma

125. A test associated with the lymph system:
a. ABGs
b. creatinine
c. DIC
d. mono test

126. Lymph fluid keeps moving in the right direction because of:
a. functioning of the lymphatic ducts
b. lymphatic capillary structure
c. pressure created by the arterial system
d. valves in the lymph vessels

127. Which is *not* a function of lymphatic nodes?
a. process lymphocytes
b. remove impurities
c. synthesize coagulation factors
d. trap and destroy bacteria

128. Which of the following veins is *not* an antecubital vein?
a. basilic
b. cephalic
c. median cubital
d. femoral

129. The ability of platelets to stick to surfaces is called platelet:
a. aggregation
b. adhesion
c. cohesion
d. inhibition

130. Which test is performed on whole blood?
a. BUN
b. CBC
c. CPK
d. protime

ANSWERS TO REVIEW QUESTIONS

1. *l.* right pulmonary arteries
2. *j.* superior vena cava
3. *g.* tricuspid valve
4. *d.* right ventricle
5. *i.* aortic valve

6. *c.* left atrium
7. *o.* left pulmonary vein
8. *a.* aortic arch
9. *c.* The heart (Fig. 5-5) has three layers: the epicardium is the thin outer

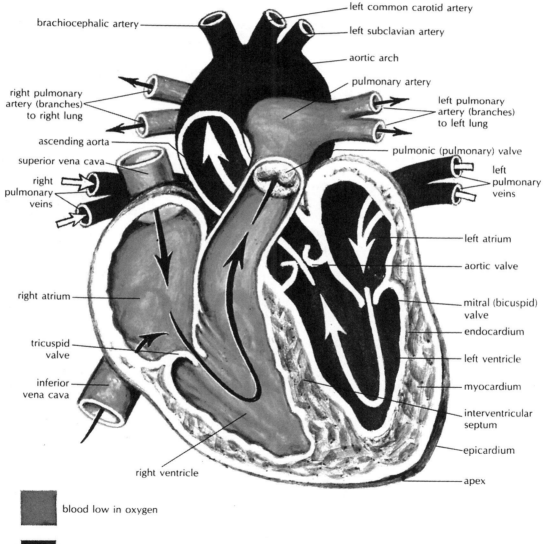

brachiocephalic artery
left common carotid artery
left subclavian artery
aortic arch
pulmonary artery
right pulmonary artery (branches) to right lung
left pulmonary artery (branches) to left lung
ascending aorta
pulmonic (pulmonary) valve
superior vena cava
left pulmonary veins
right pulmonary veins
left atrium
aortic valve
right atrium
mitral (bicuspid) valve
endocardium
tricuspid valve
left ventricle
inferior vena cava
myocardium
interventricular septum
epicardium
right ventricle
apex

blood low in oxygen

blood high in oxygen

FIGURE 5-5. Heart and great vessels.

layer; the myocardium is the thick muscular middle layer; and the endocardium is the thin membrane lining the heart. The pericardium is the double layered sac enclosing the heart.

10. **b.** The left ventricle (see Fig. 5-5) pumps oxygenated blood into the systemic circulation via the aorta. The right ventricle pumps deoxygenated blood into the pulmonary artery to be delivered to the lungs via the pulmonary circulation.

11. **d.** The heart has four chambers: the right and left atria and the right and left ventricles (see Fig 5-5).

12. **c.** Myocardial infarction or heart attack is a condition caused by occlusion of one or more of the coronary arteries which leads to ischemia or insufficient blood supply to the heart muscle. The term arrhythmia or dysrhythmia means irregularity or loss of heart rhythm. Tachycardia signifies a fast heart rate (over 100 beats per minute).

13. **a.** "Atria" is plural for atrium. The atria are the upper chambers of the heart and are called receiving chambers because they receive blood as it returns to the heart. The "chordae tendineae" are thin tissues that attach the atrioventricular valves to the walls of the ventricles to keep the valves from flipping back into the atria. The vena cavae are two large veins that deliver blood to the right atrium. The ventricles are the lower chambers of the heart that deliver blood to vessels exiting the heart.

14. **d.** The pericardium is a thin, double-layered sac enclosing the heart. The root word "cardi" means heart and the following prefixes indicate position of the layers: peri = around; epi = upon, over; myo = muscle; and endo = within.

15. **d.** Ventricles, from the Latin word "ventriculus" meaning "little belly" are the lower cavities of the heart. The atria are the upper chambers that are connected to the ventricles by valves. The septum is the partition that divides the heart into two sides, right and left.

16. **d.** The QRS complex (a collection of three waves) along with the T wave represents the electrical activity of the ventricles while the P wave represents the activity of the atria (Fig. 5-6).

17. **d.** The septum (see Fig. 5-5) is the partition that divides the heart into two sides, each side containing two chambers; an atrium and a ventricle.

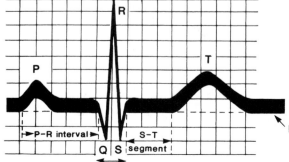

FIGURE 5-6. Normal ECG tracing showing one cardiac cycle (Jones SA, Weigel A, White RD, McSwain NE, Breiter M).

The pericardium is the membranous sac covering the heart. The chordae tendineae are thin threads of tissue that attach the valves to the walls of the ventricles to keep them from flipping back into the atria as the ventricle contracts.

18. *a.* The coronary or cardiac arteries, which are the first branches off of the aorta, furnish the blood supply to the heart. The pulmonary arteries carry blood from the right atrium to the lungs. The vena cavae deliver blood to the heart from the systemic system. Venules are the smallest branches of veins.

19. *b.* One complete contraction and subsequent relaxation of the heart is called a "cardiac cycle." The relaxing phase is called diastole while the contracting phase is called systole. A heart attack is called a cardiac infarction. Bradycardia is the term used to describe an irregular slow heart rate of less than 60 beats per minute.

20. *d.* The sinoatrial node (SA node) (Fig. 5–7) is called the heart's "pacemaker." It generates an electrical impulse which initiates the contraction of both atria pushing the blood into the ventricles. The impulse is picked up by the atrioventricular (AV) node and relayed through the bundle of His and along the Purkinje fibers throughout the ventricles, causing them to contract. The semilunar or crescent-shaped valves open as the ventricles contract to allow the blood to flow into the exit arteries.

21. *b.* The complete cardiac cycle involving the simultaneous contraction of both atria pushing the blood into the ventricles followed by the simultaneous contraction of the ventricles pushing the blood into the exit arteries and then the relaxation of both takes approximately 0.8 seconds.

22. *d.* An ECG is the actual record of electrical currents that correspond to each event in the heart muscle contraction. An electroencephalogram (EEG) measures electrical currents from the brain. Creatine kinase (CK) and arterial blood gases (ABGs) are diagnostic blood tests used to measure heart muscle damage and changes in the acid-base balance

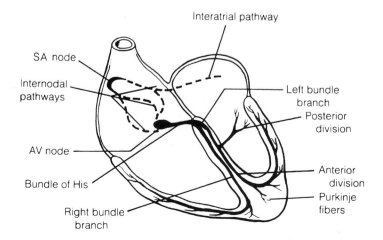

FIGURE 5-7. The electrical conduction system of the heart (Jones SA, Weigel A, White RD, McSwain NE, Breiter M).

Interatrial pathway

SA node

Internodal pathways

AV node

Bundle of His

Right bundle branch

Left bundle branch

Posterior division

Anterior division

Purkinje fibers

of blood, respectively (see Fig. 5-6).

23. *a.* The P wave represents the activity of the atria and is usually the first wave seen. The QRS complex along with the T wave represents the activity of the ventricles (see Fig. 5-6).

24. *d.* The right atrioventricular valve (AV valve) found between the right atrium and ventricle is also called the tricuspid valve because it has three flaps or cusps. The bicuspid valve or left AV has two cusps and is also called the mitral valve. The pulmonary valve (right semilunar valve) is so named because it allows blood to pass into the pulmonary artery from the right ventricle (see Fig. 5-5).

25. *d.* Murmurs are abnormal heart sounds, usually caused by faulty valve action. Extrasystoles, fibrillations, and arrhythmias are abnormal contractions, not sounds.

26. *a.* An artery is a vessel that carries blood away from the heart. Veins, such as the vena cava, carry blood to the heart. Capillaries are vessels that connect the ends of the smallest arteries (arterioles) to the smallest veins (venules).

27. *c.* The wave of increased pressure created as the ventricles contract and blood is forced out of the heart through the arteries creates the throbbing beat known as the pulse.

28. *d.* Unlike the arterial system, veins do not have sufficient pressure from the heart's contractions to keep the blood moving through them. Veins rely on skeletal muscle movement around them and the opening and closing of the valves to keep the blood moving toward the heart.

29. *d.* All of the answers deal with heart rates or rhythm. Tachycardia is an

abnormally fast rate. Bradycardia is a slow rate. Extrasystole is the term for an extra beat before the normal beat. Fibrillation is the term for rapid, uncoordinated contractions.

30. *d.* Blood pressure is a measure of the pressure exerted on the walls of a blood vessel. It is commonly measured in a large artery, such as the brachial. Blood pressure is expressed in millimeters of mercury and has two components: the systolic pressure which is the highest pressure reached during ventricular contraction, and the diastolic pressure which occurs during relaxation of the ventricles. Systolic pressure for the normal, relaxed, sitting adult averages 120 mm Hg while diastolic averages 80 mm Hg.

31. *c.* The word "endocarditis" means inflammation of the endocardium. The endocardium is the thin membrane lining the inner surface of the heart. Pericarditis is inflammation of the pericardium which is the thin, fluid-filled sac that surrounds the heart. Angina pectoris refers to pain in the area of the heart caused by decreased blood flow to the muscle layer of the heart. Aortic stenosis is the term used to describe a narrowing of the aorta or its opening.

32. *c.* CPK (CK) and LDH are enzymes present in cardiac muscle. They are released during myocardial infarction. Alkaline phosphatase and SGPT are enzymes measured most commonly to determine liver function. Blood urea nitrogen (BUN) is a kidney function test and prothrombin time (PT) is a coagulation test used to monitor anticoagulant therapy. A glucose tolerance test (GTT) measures

glucose metabolism and erythrocyte sedimentation rate (ESR) is a nonspecific indicator of disease, especially inflammatory conditions such as arthritis.

33. **b.** Systolic pressure is the pressure in the arteries during contraction of the ventricles. Diastolic pressure is the arterial pressure when the ventricles are relaxed. Because the atrial contraction is so very close to the ventricle contraction, blood pressure for atrial contraction cannot easily be detected and is not normally measured.

34. **a.** Pulmonary circulation carries deoxygenated blood from the right ventricle of the heart to the lungs via the pulmonary artery. It also returns oxygenated blood from the lungs to the left atrium of the heart via the pulmonary vein. The left ventricle pumps the oxygenated blood into the arterial systemic circulation via the aorta. The arterial systemic circulation delivers the blood to the tissues. The venous systemic circulation returns deoxygenated blood to the heart (Fig. 5-8).

35. **b.** Because it is full of oxygen, normal systemic arterial blood is bright cherry red in color. Normal systemic venous blood is dark red with a bluish tinge. Regardless of what some people think, no one has blue blood.

36. **a.** The aorta, at the start of the systemic arterial circulation, is the largest artery in the body. The

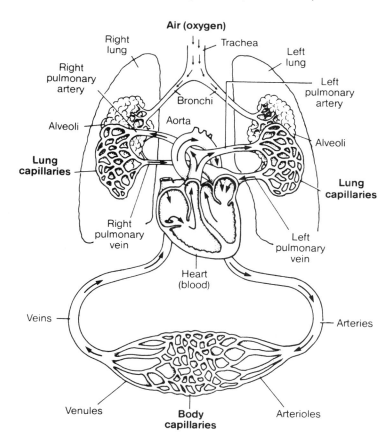

FIGURE 5-8. Representation of the vascular flow (National Tuberculosis and Respiratory Disease Association, New York, NY).

largest vein in the body is the vena cava. The femoral artery is a large artery in the leg. The carotid artery is a large artery in the neck.

37. *c.* The pulmonary vein carries oxygenated blood from the lungs to the heart. All vessels that return blood to the heart are called veins. All vessels that carry blood away from the heart are called arteries. The general "rule of thumb" that all arteries carry oxygenated blood is only true for the systemic circulation. In the pulmonary circulation, the vessel that carries oxygenated blood from the lungs is called a vein because it is returning the blood to the heart. The vessel that carries deoxygenated blood to the lungs is called the pulmonary artery because it is carrying the blood away from the heart.

38. *a.* Sphygmomanometer is the technical name for a blood pressure cuff. An electrocardiogram (ECG) is a record (tracing) of the electrical activity of the heart. A machine that records brain waves is used in electroencephalography (EEG). A pacemaker is an electrical device that automatically generates electrical impulses to initiate the heart beat.

39. *d.* The smallest veins are called venules. Arterioles are the smallest arteries. Capillaries connect the arterioles, which are the end of the arterial system, to the venules which are the beginning of venous system. Lumen is the term for the internal space of any vessel.

40. *c.* The pulmonary artery, as its name infers, is part of the pulmonary circulation. The brachial artery, cephalic vein, and vena cava are all part of the systemic circulation.

41. *c.* The saphenous vein runs the entire length of the leg and is considered the longest vein in the body. The largest vein and artery in the body are, respectively, the vena cava and the aorta. There is a femoral vein and a femoral artery. Both are located in the leg (see Fig. 5-9).

42. *b.* Capillaries are tiny one-cell-thick vessels that form the fine network that delivers oxygen and nutrients to the tissues and carries carbon dioxide and other waste products away. Arterioles and venules, on the other hand, have multiple layers like arteries and veins. The vena cava, the largest vein in the body, also has multiple layers.

43. *b.* The pulmonary vein is part of the pulmonary circulation and carries oxygenated blood from the lungs to the heart so that it can be pumped to the body. The superior vena cava and the brachial vein are part of the systemic venous circulation and carry deoxygenated blood back to the heart. The pulmonary artery carries deoxygenated blood from the heart to the lungs.

44. *a.* The tunica adventitia is the term applied to the outer layer of an artery or vein. It is made up of connective tissue and is thicker in arteries than veins. The tunica media is the middle layer, composed of smooth muscle and some elastic fibers. The tunica media is much thicker in arteries than in veins. The tunica intima, sometimes also called tunica interna, is the inner layer or lining of a blood vessel and is composed of a single layer of endothelial cells with an underlying basement membrane, connective tissue layer, and elastic membrane.

45. *b.* The space within a blood vessel is called the lumen. The tunica intima and tunica media are blood vessel layers. The endothelium is the inner lining of a blood vessel.

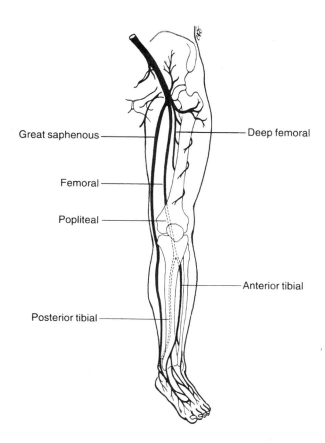

Great saphenous

Deep femoral

Femoral

Popliteal

Anterior tibial

Posterior tibial

FIGURE 5-9. Major leg and foot veins.

46. **d.** The smooth muscle of the tunica media is much thicker in arteries than in veins. The tunica adventitia or outer layer is also thicker in arteries. Both veins and arteries are lined with a single layer of endothelial cells (Fig. 5-10).

47. **c.** You can tell the structure in Figure 5-2 is a vein because it has a valve. Arteries do not have valves.

48. **b.** Blood flows from the heart into arteries which branch into smaller and smaller arteries, the smallest of which are called arterioles. Arterioles connect with capillaries which in turn are connected to the smallest veins which are called venules. Blood from the arterioles passes through the capillaries where the exchange of gases, nutrients, and waste products takes place. From the capillaries the blood flows into the venules which merge with larger and larger veins until the blood returns to the heart. Choices "a" and "c" are obviously incorrect. In choice "d" the blood would be traveling the wrong direction (see Fig. 5-8).

49. **c.** The inner layer of a blood vessel is called the tunica intima. The lumen is the internal space within a blood vessel. The tunica adventitia and media are the outside layer and middle layer, respectively (see Fig. 5-10).

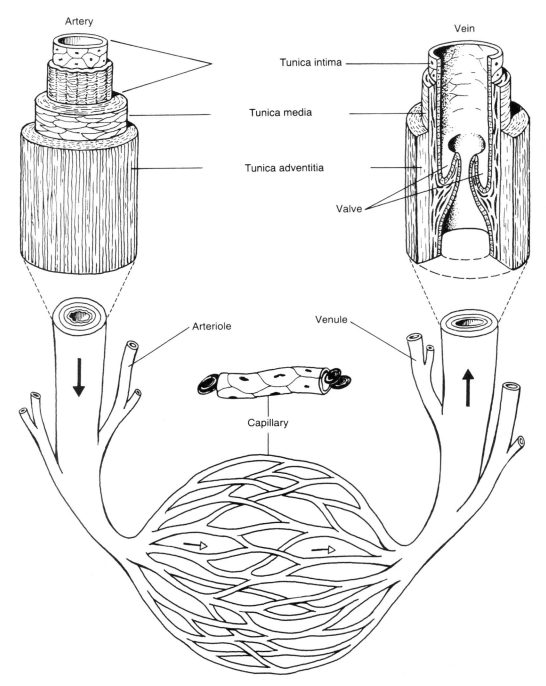

FIGURE 5-10. Artery, vein, and capillary structure.

50. *a.* The left ventricle delivers blood to the aorta. The left atrium delivers blood to the left ventricle. The pulmonary artery delivers blood from the right ventricle to the lungs. The pulmonary vein returns blood from the lungs to the heart (see Fig. 5-8).

51. *d.* In choosing the best vein, the first selection is the median cubital because it is large, bruises less easily, and is well anchored. The cephalic vein is the next choice because it is better anchored and less painful to puncture than the basilic. The basilic vein is the last choice because it rolls easily and there is the possibility of accidentally puncturing the brachial artery and a major nerve when this vein is used (see Fig. 5-3).

52. *c.* Capillaries are the smallest blood vessels. They are one-cell-thick which allows for the exchange of oxygen and nutrients between the cells and the blood. Alveoli are thin-walled saclike chambers within the lungs where oxygen and carbon dioxide are exchanged between the air and blood. Arterioles are tiny arteries that connect with and deliver blood to the capillaries. Venules are tiny veins at the junction where the capillaries merge with the venous circulation.

53. *a.* The antecubital fossa is located in front of (anterior) and below (distal) to the elbow.

54. *c.* A blood clot or part of a blood clot circulating in the bloodstream is called an embolus. An aneurism is a bulging or dilation of a blood vessel. An embolism is the obstruction of a blood vessel by a blood clot or other undissolved matter. A thrombus is a stationary blood clot that obstructs a blood vessel.

55. *c.* cephalic

56. *d.* median cubital

57. *a.* basilic

58. *d.* The basilic vein is the third choice of veins in the antecubital fossa area for all of the reasons listed.

59. *b.* Ankle and foot veins should *never* be punctured routinely. They are used only when no other suitable sites are available *and* the patient's physician has given permission to do so. Coagulation problems and poor circulation may cause serious problems as well as erroneous results when ankle or foot veins are used.

60. *a.* Blood is a mixture of fluid and cells. The fluid portion is called *plasma*. Plasma is approximately 90% water and 10% dissolved substances such as antibodies, nutrients, minerals, and gases. Red blood cells (erythrocytes), and platelets are part of the cellular portion of blood referred to as the *formed elements*. Bacteria are not normally found in the blood.

61. *c.* Phlebitis is the medical term for vein inflammation. An embolism is the obstruction of a blood vessel by a blood clot or other undissolved foreign matter. Hemostasis is the process by which bleeding is stopped. Thrombosis means the formation or existence of a blood clot in the vascular system.

62. *c.* A disseminated intravascular coagulation (DIC) screen is a series of tests to detect diffuse uncontrolled coagulation throughout the vascular system. In DIC situations, continuous generation of thrombin causes depletion of several clotting factors to such an extent that generalized bleeding may occur.

Bilirubin is a liver function test. Glucose is a test of carbohydrate metabolism. A cerebrospinal fluid (CSF) test is considered a nervous system test.

63. *a.* Atherosclerosis is a form of arteriosclerosis involving changes in the intima of the artery caused by the accumulation of lipid material. Blood cholesterol levels when increased constitute an increased risk of developing coronary heart disease. Endocarditis means inflammation of the lining membrane of the heart and may be caused by invasion of microorganisms. Phlebitis means inflammation of a vein.

64. *a.* An aneurysm is a localized dilation or bulging of a blood vessel, usually an artery. An embolism is the obstruction of a blood vessel by a blood clot or other undissolved foreign matter. Arteriosclerosis is a hardening or thickening and loss of elasticity of the wall of the artery. Thrombophlebitis is defined as inflammation of the vein in conjunction with the formation of a blood clot.

65. *c.* Thrombophlebitis is defined as inflammation of a vein in conjunction with the formation of a blood clot. Vasculitis is a general term meaning inflammation of a blood vessel. Phlebitis is more specific and means vein inflammation. Phlebitis can lead to thrombophlebitis. Sclerosis when pertaining to the vascular system refers to a thickening or hardening of the wall of a blood vessel.

66. *c.* The average 154-lb adult has approximately 5 L or 5.2 qt of blood. More exact blood volume can be calculated based on the fact that the average adult has 70 mL of blood per each kilogram of weight.

67. *c.* The normal ratio of plasma to formed elements is approximately 55% plasma and 45% cells. When estimating how much serum or plasma will be available for testing most laboratorians usually figure that approximately half of a normal blood specimen will be serum or plasma.

68. *b.* Normal plasma is a clear, pale yellow fluid that is 90% water.

69. *c.* "A hand in pronation" means the palm of the hand faces downward, thus causing the cephalic vein to be in line with the little finger.

70. *b.* The type of cell that is most numerous in the blood is the erythrocyte or red blood cell averaging 4.5 to 5.0 million per cubic millimeter of blood.

71. *b.* All mature leukocytes or white blood cells contain nuclei. Thrombocytes (platelets) and mature erythrocytes (red blood cells) do not have a nucleus. A reticulocyte is an immature red blood cell that contains remnants of nuclear material, but not a complete nucleus (see Fig. 5-11).

72. *c.* Reticulocytes are immature red blood cells in the bloodstream that contain nuclear remnants.

73. *a.* The granulocytes called eosinophils (eos) are increased in allergic reactions and parasitic infestations such as a case of pinworms. Eos ingest and detoxify foreign protein and help turn off immune reactions.

74. *b.* Normal erythrocytes are described as anuclear, biconcave disks approximately 7 μm to 8 μm in diameter.

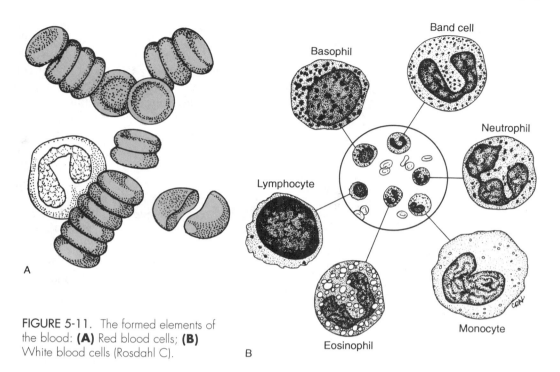

FIGURE 5-11. The formed elements of the blood: **(A)** Red blood cells; **(B)** White blood cells (Rosdahl C).

75. *b.* Leukocytes (white blood cells) are produced in the bone marrow and lymphatic tissue.

76. *d.* The primary function of red blood cells is to transport oxygen from the lungs to the tissues. A secondary function of red blood cells is to transport carbon dioxide from the tissues to the lungs. Nutrients and antibodies are not transported by red blood cells but are carried dissolved in the plasma.

77. *d.* Leukocyte is the medical term for a white blood cell.

78. *b.* Leukocytes have the ability to pass through the walls of blood vessels. They are said to have extravascular function, which means they do their job outside the blood stream. Erythrocytes, reticulocytes, and platelets have intravascular function and cannot pass through intact blood vessel walls.

79. *b.* Neutrophils are a type of leukocyte that are able to destroy bacteria and small particles by a process called phagocytosis.

80. *d.* The term "polys" comes from the word polymorphonuclear. Neutrophils are sometimes called polys because they have a nucleus with several lobes.

81. *a.* The first cell on the scene when an injury occurs is the platelet. The role of the platelet is to aggregate with other platelets and adhere to injured area thus forming a platelet plug.

82. *a.* Erythrocytes or red blood cells are described as anuclear (non-nucleated), biconcave disks approximately 7 μm to 8 μm in diameter (see Fig. 5-11).

83. *d.* Monocytes that have left the bloodstream are sometimes referred to as macrophages because they are found in the loose connective tissue where they phagocytize particles much like cells of the R.E. system.

84. *b.* A type of lymphocyte called a B-lymphocyte differentiates into a plasma cell.

85. *c.* A typical neutrophil is polymorphonuclear meaning it has a nucleus with several lobes or segments. Thus, the natural tendency is to call this cell a "seg" (see Fig. 5-11).

86. *d.* Thrombo/cyte when separated into word parts means clotting/cell and is a another medical term for platelet.

87. *c.* A platelet is not a true cell but a cytoplasmic fragment of a large bone marrow cell called a mega/karyo/cyte, a term which when separated into word parts means large/nucleated/cell.

88. *d.* An individual's blood type is inherited and is determined by the presence or absence of certain types of antigens on the surface of the red blood cells. The ABO blood group system recognizes four blood types based on two antigens called A and B. A type A individual has the A antigen; type B has the B antigen; type AB has both antigens; and type O has neither A nor B. The Rh system is based on the presence or absence of the Rh antigen. An Rh-positive individual has the Rh antigen and an Rh-negative individual lacks the Rh antigen.

89. *b.* To prevent sensitization from an Rh+ fetus, an Rh− woman may be given Rh immunoglobulin at certain times during her pregnancy, as well as immediately after the baby's birth. Rh immunoglobulin will destroy any Rh+ fetal cells that may have entered her bloodstream thus preventing sensitization. Only an Rh-negative person can become sensitized to the Rh factor.

90. *c.* Becoming sensitized means that the individual may produce antibodies against the Rh factor. Rh antibodies produced by the mother can cross the placenta into the fetal circulation and cause the destruction of red blood cells of a subsequent Rh+ fetus.

91. *a.* An individual whose blood type is A positive has red blood cells that have the A antigen but lack the Rh antigen. (See answer to question 88.)

92. *d.* Hemolytic disease of the newborn is most often the result of an Rh− mother being sensitized by a previous Rh+ fetus causing her to form Rh antibodies. During a subsequent pregnancy these antibodies can cross the placenta into the fetal circulation and attack the red blood cells of the fetus and cause hemolysis.

93. *b.* Whole blood like the blood found in the body is made up of a liquid portion called plasma which contains formed elements, red blood cells, white blood cells, and platelets suspended in it.

94. *d.* Clotted blood is made up of two parts, a clotted portion containing cells enmeshed in fibrin and a liquid portion called serum.

95. *b.* After centrifugation of whole blood, the liquid portion called plasma is at the top of the tube and the cellular portion is at the bottom.

96. *a.* The arrow in Figure 5-4 points to the layer of white blood cells and platelets called the buffy coat.

97. *d.* You cannot visually tell serum from plasma because both serum and plasma are clear, pale yellow fluids.

98. *c.* EDTA is the anticoagulant of choice for hematology studies. However, if a blood smear is to be made from an EDTA specimen, it should be made within 1 hour of collection because prolonged contact with EDTA may change the staining characteristics of the formed elements.

99. *c.* The most common anticoagulants are EDTA, sodium citrate, and heparin. EDTA and sodium citrate prevent coagulation by binding calcium into a calcium salt. Without calcium ions, the coagulation process cannot take place. Heparin inhibits thrombin. Without thrombin, the blood cannot form a fibrin clot.

100. *b.* Most chemistry tests are ideally performed on serum because nothing has to be added to the blood during collection. Unfortunately, to obtain serum, a normal blood specimen must be allowed to clot for at least 20 to 30 minutes before being centrifuged. With the exception of fibrinogen, plasma contains the same analytes as serum but because a plasma specimen does not clot it can be spun immediately after collection and tested 20 to 30 minutes sooner. A fast turn around time is vitally important for stat requests.

101. *a.* Bleeding time tests assess the ability of the platelet to aggregate (degranulate and stick to one another) and form a platelet plug.

FDP, PT, and PTT test other parts of the coagulation process.

102. *b.* To obtain serum, blood must be allowed to clot. During the clotting process, fibrinogen is split into fibrin which enmeshes the cells and forms a clot. Once the clotting is complete the specimen is centrifuged and the clear liquid obtained is called serum. Serum does not contain fibrinogen because it was used up in the clotting process.

103. *c.* The word "thrombo/cyt/osis" means clotting/cell/condition. The term is used to describe a condition in which the clotting cells (platelets) are abnormally increased.

104. *a.* Anemia is a blood disorder usually characterized by an abnormal reduction in the number of red blood cells in the circulating blood. Leukopenia is characterized by abnormally decreased white blood cells. Thrombocytopenia is abnormally decreased platelets. Polycythemia is overproduction of red blood cells.

105. *c.* The process of coagulation which means stopping or controlling the flow of blood is also called hemostasis. Hemoconcentration means increased nonfilterable elements. Hemolysis is destruction of red blood cells. Homeostasis is the state of equilibrium or balance the body strives to maintain.

106. *b.* Assessing the formed elements, red blood cells, white blood cells, and platelets, is part of a complete blood count (CBC). It is performed on whole blood. BUN, electrolytes, and glucose are chemistry tests performed on serum or plasma.

107. *d.* Hemo/stasis means blood/stopping or controlling and refers to the process of coagulation.

108. *b.* Leuko/cyt/osis means white/cell/condition. The term is used to describe an abnormal increase of white blood cells.

109. *a.* The ion (particle carrying an electrical charge) necessary to convert prothrombin to thrombin in the coagulation cascade is calcium (Ca+).

110. *d.* The word extrinsic means "from or coming from, without." The extrinsic pathway is initiated by tissue injury, causing the release of thromboplastin (factor III) and the activation of factor VII. The intrinsic pathway of coagulation is initiated by events within the bloodstream. Factor VIII (antihemophilic factor) is part of the intrinsic pathway. Platelet plug formation is the second stage in the coagulation process and occurs before the initiation of either pathway.

111. *d.* There are four stages to the hemostasis process, the initial stage is the constriction of vessels (vasoconstriction) to slow down blood loss. The second stage is platelet plug formation, which involves platelet aggregation and adhesion. These first two stages are called primary hemostasis. Stage three is fibrin clot formation which involves the activation of the intrinsic and extrinsic pathways of the coagulation cascade. Stage four is fibrinolysis, the process by which the fibrin clot is dissolved.

112. *b.* Both complete blood count and hemoglobin are hematology tests used to assess blood disorders. Ferritin is the form in which iron is stored in the tissues. It is a whole blood test performed in chemistry that is also used in the diagnoses of blood disorders. Creatinine is a kidney function test performed in the chemistry department.

113. *d.* The word primary means first. The first two stages of the hemostasis/coagulation process are vasoconstriction and platelet plug formation. These first two stages combined are called primary hemostasis and are sometimes all that is needed to stop blood loss and the process goes no further.

114. *b.* Lymph fluid is similar to plasma but is 95% water instead of 90%. Unlike serum, lymph does contain fibrinogen. It is unlike urine or whole blood.

115. *b.* Hemophilia is an hereditary blood disorder characterized by very long bleeding times. The most common type of hemophilia is caused by the lack of factor VIII.

116. *b.* The liver plays a major role in coagulation. It synthesizes the clotting factors fibrinogen and prothrombin and is the source of heparin, a naturally formed anticoagulant found in the bloodstream.

117. *b.* The last stage of the coagulation process is called fibrinolysis. In this stage the protein plasminogen is converted to the enzyme, plasmin, whose purpose is to split fibrin into small fragments called FDP which are then removed by phagocytic cells of the reticuloendothelial system.

118. *b.* Tests used to evaluate primary hemostasis or platelet plug formation, are platelet count and

bleeding time. The other choices are tests that measure the functioning of secondary hemostasis.

119. *b.* Obstruction of a blood vessel by an embolus causes an embolism.

120. *d.* A PT or prothrombin test (protime) is a coagulation test. Electrolytes are a chemistry test. Glycohemoglobin is a chemistry test that measures glucose bound to hemoglobin. Hemoglobin is a hematology test.

121. *c.* The anatomical position refers to the body as if the patient is standing erect, arms at the side with palms facing forward. In this position, the basilic vein is on the same side as the little finger.

122. *a.* Body cells are nourished from the tissue fluid acquired from the bloodstream. Much of the fluid diffuses back into the capillaries along with waste products of metabolism. Excess tissue fluid filters into lymphatic capillaries, where it is called lymph.

123. *c.* Stage 1, vasoconstriction, and stage 2, platelet plug formation, are referred to as primary hemostasis. Normally a needle puncture of a vein can be healed through primary hemostasis alone.

124. *d.* The word parts, lympho/sarc/oma combine to mean lymphoid/ fleshy/malignant tumor.

125. *d.* The test most often associated with the lymph system is mononucleosis which is an acute infectious disease that primarily affects lymphoid tissue.

126. *d.* The lymph fluid moves through the lymph vessels primarily by skeletal muscle contraction much like blood moves through the veins. Like veins, the lymph vessels have valves to keep the lymph flowing in the right direction.

127. *c.* The lymph nodes function to remove impurities, produce lymphocytes, and trap and destroy impurities. Lymph nodes *do not* synthesize coagulation factors.

128. *d.* The femoral vein is found in the upper portion of the leg and is a continuation of the popliteal vein. The basilic, cephalic, and median cubital are antecubital veins.

129. *b.* The word adhesion means "the uniting of two surfaces or parts," as in platelet adhesion to the injured area. The ability of platelets to stick to one another is called platelet aggregation.

130. *b.* To perform hematology tests, such as a complete blood count, the specimen must be whole blood. This allows the laboratory technologist to look at and count the cells in suspension as they are in the body.

Infection Control, Safety, and First Aid

II. Safety

A. General Laboratory Safety Rules
B. Safety Rules in Patient Rooms and Other Areas
C. Biological Hazards
   1. Definition
   2. Routes of Entry
      a. Ingestion
      b. Parenteral
         (1) Non-Intact Skin
         (2) Percutaneous
         (3) Mucous Membrane
      c. Airborne
   3. Occupational Exposure
   4. Exposure Incident Procedures
   5. Exposure Control Plan
      a. Exposure Determination
      b. Methods of Implementation
         (1) Universal Precautions Statement
         (2) Engineering Controls
         (3) Work Practice Controls
         (4) Personal Protective Equipment (PPE)
         (5) Housekeeping Schedule and Methods
      c. Hepatitis B Vaccine
      d. Communication of Hazards to Employees
         (1) Warning Labels
         (2) Training and Information
      e. Record Keeping
         (1) Medical Records
         (2) Training Records
D. Electrical Safety
   1. Guidelines
   2. Actions to Take if Electrical Shock Occurs
E. Fire Safety
   1. Components of Fire
   2. Classes of Fire
   3. Fire Extinguishers
   4. Fire Safety Do's and Don'ts
   5. National Fire Protection Association (NFPA)
F. Radiation Safety
   1. Principles
   2. Hazards
G. Chemical Safety
   1. Guidelines
   2. Chemical Identification
      a. OSHA Hazardous Communications (HAZCOM) Standard
      b. National Fire Protection Association (NFPA)
      c. Material Safety Data Sheets (MSDS)
      d. Department of Transportation (DOT)
      e. Environmental Protection Agency (EPA)
   3. Safety Showers and Eyewash stations
   4. Chemical Spills

III. First Aid

A. External Hemorrhage
B. Shock Prevention
   1. Common Symptoms of Shock
   2. First Aid for Shock
C. Cardiopulmonary Resuscitation

REVIEW QUESTIONS

1. Which of the following is proper neonatal ICU blood drawing procedure?
   a. keep your blood drawing tray as close to the isolette as possible
   b. never awaken an infant to draw blood
   c. use povidone-iodine to clean a skin puncture site
   d. wear mask, gown, and gloves

2. What does the NFPA codeword *RACE* mean?

a. rescue, alarm, confine, extinguish
b. rescue, activate, cover, extinguish
c. run, alarm, counter, extinguish
d. run, activate, confine, escape

3. Which of the following statements concerning an employee blood-borne pathogen exposure incident is *not necessarily* true?
   a. all exposure incidents should be reported to a supervisor
   b. an exposed employee should have access to a free confidential medical evaluation
   c. the exposure should be documented on an incident report form
   d. the source patient must submit to HIV and HBV testing

4. When the chain of infection is broken:
   a. an individual becomes immune
   b. an individual becomes susceptible
   c. infection is prevented
   d. infection results

5. Considering all patients to be potentially infectious for hepatitis or HIV is the concept of:
   a. disease-specific isolation
   b. isolation techniques
   c. infection control
   d. universal precautions

6. Which organization helps establish regulations and guidelines for infection control?
   a. CDC
   b. JCAHO
   c. OSHA
   d. all the above

7. Which type of isolation would be used for a patient who has active TB?
   a. contact
   b. enteric
   c. respiratory or AFB
   d. reverse

8. Which of the following is *not* recommended by the OSHA Blood-borne Pathogen Standard?

a. dismissal of HIV-positive workers
b. handwashing following glove removal
c. HBV immunization
d. use of protective barriers

9. The virus that causes AIDS is:
   a. HAV
   b. HBV
   c. HIV
   d. none of the above

10. A person who has recovered from a particular virus and has developed antibodies against a particular virus is said to be:
    a. a carrier
    b. immune
    c. infectious
    d. susceptible

11. According to standard first aid procedures, severe external bleeding is *best* controlled by:
    a. application of direct pressure and elevation of the extremity
    b. applying a tourniquet
    c. keeping the injured extremity below the level of the heart
    d. raising the victim's head above the level of the injury

12. The main purpose of an infection control program is to:
    a. determine the source of communicable infections
    b. isolate infectious patients from other patients
    c. prevent the spread of infection in the hospital
    d. protect patients from outside contamination

13. A pathogen is:
    a. a communicable virus
    b. an organism capable of causing disease
    c. any microorganism
    d. normal flora of the skin

14. Which disease does *not* involve a blood-borne pathogen?
    a. hepatitis B
    b. hepatitis C
    c. HIV infection
    d. tuberculosis

15. Which is *not* proper handwashing procedure?
    a. stand back so that clothing does not touch the sink
    b. wet hands with water before applying soap
    c. wash for at least 15 seconds
    d. turn the faucet off with the towel used to dry your hands

16. An example of a disease requiring respiratory isolation:
    a. chicken pox
    b. influenza
    c. pertussis
    d. *Shigella*

17. A Class C fire:
    a. involves combustible metals
    b. involves electrical equipment
    c. involves flammable liquids
    d. occurs with ordinary materials

18. Universal precautions should be followed:
    a. if a patient is in isolation
    b. when a patient is known to be HIV positive
    c. when a patient is known to have HBV
    d. with all patients, at all times

19. Vaccination against HBV involves:
    a. a dose of vaccine, another 1 month later, and a final dose 6 months later
    b. a single dose of vaccine that confers lifetime immunity
    c. three doses of vaccine, each 3 months apart, then yearly doses thereafter
    d. there is no vaccine for HBV

20. Objects capable of adhering to infectious material and transmitting disease are called:
    a. fomites
    b. vectors
    c. vehicles
    d. none of the above

21. The "right to know" law primarily deals with:
    a. electrical safety
    b. first aid procedures
    c. hazardous materials information
    d. universal precautions

22. How would a phlebotomist know which precautions to use for category-specific isolation?
    a. ask the patient's nurse
    b. follow the instructions on the card on the door
    c. no special precautions are required for category-specific isolation
    d. wear a gown, gloves, and mask just to be safe

23. Strict isolation is used for patients with:
    a. highly contagious diseases
    b. respiratory infections
    c. severe burns
    d. surgical wounds

24. The body organ targeted by HBV is:
    a. brain
    b. heart
    c. liver
    d. lungs

25. The three components of fire referred to as the fire triangle are:
    a. combustible material, carbon dioxide, heat
    b. fuel, oxygen, heat
    c. fuel, oxygen, static electricity
    d. vapor, carbon dioxide, energy

26. Which of the following are means of breaking the chain of infection?
    a. handwashing and glove use
    b. isolation procedures

c. stress reduction and proper nutrition
d. all the above

27. What is the proper way to dispose of laboratory specimens and contaminated supplies, other than sharps, when following BSI?
    a. double bag and throw in the trash
    b. place in labeled biohazard bags or containers
    c. place in puncture-resistant containers
    d. throw in trash that is to be incinerated

28. Which of the following is *not* improper electrical safety procedure?
    a. handling electrical equipment with wet hands
    b. using frayed electrical cords
    c. using extension cords when necessary
    d. servicing electrical equipment when unplugged

29. According to the American Heart Association, the first thing to do before initiating cardiopulmonary resuscitation (CPR) is to:
    a. open airway
    b. check breathing
    c. check circulation
    d. check responsiveness

30. Which isolation system requires wearing of gloves when contacting or handling *any* body fluid?
    a. body substance isolation
    b. disease-specific isolation
    c. enteric isolation
    d. universal precautions

31. Protocol when entering respiratory isolation requires the phlebotomist to wear:
    a. a gown
    b. a mask
    c. eye protection
    d. gloves

32. The majority of exposures to HIV in health care settings occur:

a. during surgery
b. from blood transfusion
c. from needlesticks
d. when touching patients with AIDS

33. Which of the following is the most common type of nosocomial infection in the United States?
    a. hepatitis infection
    b. respiratory infection
    c. urinary tract infection
    d. wound infection

34. Which of the following organizations instituted and enforces the Blood-borne Pathogen Standard?
    a. CAP
    b. CDC
    c. JCAHO
    d. OSHA

35. Which is *not* a proper laboratory safety procedure?
    a. secure long hair away from the face
    b. never eat, drink, or apply makeup in the laboratory
    c. wear closed toe shoes
    d. wear your laboratory coat at all times

36. You accidentally splash hydrochloric acid in your eye while adding it to a 24-hour urine container. What should you do first?
    a. dry your eyes with a paper towel
    b. flush your eyes with water for a minimum of 15 minutes
    c. proceed to the emergency room as quickly as possible
    d. put 10–20 drops of saline in your eyes

37. What should a phlebotomist do with the used gown when leaving strict isolation?
    a. dispose of it in a container in the laboratory
    b. fold it inside out and leave it in a proper container in the room
    c. take it off and dispose of it outside of the room
    d. throw it in the laundry at the nurses station

38. An example of employee screening for infection control:
    a. PPD testing
    b. HBV vaccination
    c. measles vaccination
    d. shot of immune globulin

39. Which type of infection transmission occurs from touching contaminated bed linens?
    a. direct contact
    b. droplet contact
    c. indirect contact
    d. vehicle contact

40. Which of the following is *not* transmitted through blood transfusion?
    a. diabetes mellitus
    b. HBV
    c. HIV
    d. syphilis

41. Which of the following is required under universal precautions?
    a. isolate HIV-positive patients
    b. label specimens from HIV-positive patients
    c. wear a mask
    d. wear gloves when performing phlebotomy procedures

42. What is the meaning of the symbol ☡ in Figure 6-1?
    a. biohazard
    b. flammable
    c. radiation hazard
    d. water reactive

43. What type of isolation would be used for a patient who has a very low white count?
    a. enteric
    b. neutropenic
    c. respiratory
    d. strict

44. What should the phlebotomist do if the outside of a patient specimen tube has blood on it?

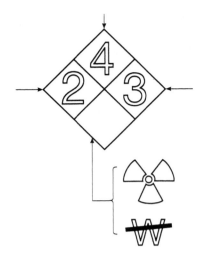

FIGURE 6-1. National Fire Protection Association diagram (Jones SA, Weigel A, White RD, McSwain NE, Breiter M).

a. discard it after pouring the contents into a clean tube
b. discard it in the patient's room and draw a new tube
c. place a biohazard label on it
d. wipe it with disinfectant

45. What does a stop sign on a patient's door signify?
    a. anyone going into the room must check with the patient's nurse before entering
    b. only hospital personnel are allowed into the room
    c. put on a gown and mask before entering
    d. visitors are not allowed in the room

46. Which of the following conditions *would not necessarily* lead to work restrictions for a hospital employee?
    a. a positive PPD test
    b. influenza
    c. rubella
    d. weeping dermatitis

47. How many classes of fire are identified by the NFPA?
   a. two
   b. three
   c. four
   d. six

48. What is the *best* means of preventing nosocomial infection?
   a. isolation procedures
   b. proper handwashing
   c. proper immunization
   d. wearing gloves

49. The purpose of "protective" isolation is to:
   a. prevent airborne transmission of disease
   b. protect others from patients with transmissible diseases
   c. protect susceptible patients from outside contamination
   d. provide a safe environment for psychiatric patients

50. An example of possible "percutaneous" infection transmission is:
   a. getting stuck with a contaminated needle
   b. handling blood specimens with ungloved badly chapped hands
   c. ingesting infectious material
   d. mucous membrane contact with infectious material

51. In which instance could an electrical shock to a patient most likely occur?
   a. drawing a patient's blood during an electrical storm
   b. drawing a patient's blood while standing in a puddle of water
   c. drawing blood from a patient who is talking on the telephone
   d. touching electrical equipment while drawing a patient's blood

52. The OSHA HAZCOM Standard is also commonly called the:

53. The *best* course of action when entering an isolation room is:
   a. follow the directions from the sign on the door
   b. wear gown, mask, and gloves
   c. wear only a gown
   d. wear only a mask

54. Which of the following is a blood-borne pathogen?
   a. influenza
   b. rubella
   c. syphilis
   d. tuberculosis

55. The degree to which an organism is capable of causing disease is called:
   a. chain of infection
   b. susceptibility
   c. viability
   d. virulence

56. Any material or substance harmful to health is a/an:
   a. biohazard
   b. chemical hazard
   c. occupational exposure
   d. pathogen

57. What is the proper order for putting on protective clothing?
   a. gloves first, then gown, mask last
   b. gown first, then gloves, mask last
   c. gown first, then mask, gloves last
   d. mask first, then gown, gloves last

58. The blue quadrant of the NFPA diamond-shaped symbol for hazardous materials indicates:
   a. fire hazard
   b. health hazard
   c. reactivity hazard
   d. specific hazard

(continued from question 52)
   a. "disclosure" law
   b. MSDS Act
   c. "Right to Know" law
   d. United Nations Placard Recognition System

59. Which labeling system uses a diamond-shaped sign containing the United Nations hazard class number and a symbol representing the hazard?
    a. CDC
    b. DOT
    c. NFPA
    d. OSHA

60. Which of the following is an unacceptable chemical safety procedure?
    a. adding acid to water
    b. familiarizing oneself with the MSDS of a new reagent
    c. mixing bleach with other cleaners
    d. reporting a malfunctioning eye-wash station to the proper authority

61. Federal law requires that hepatitis B vaccination be made available to employees assigned to duties with occupational exposure risk:
    a. immediately
    b. once their probationary employment period has ended
    c. within 1 month of employment
    d. within 10 working days of initial assignment

62. What is the *first* thing the phlebotomist should do in the event of an accidental needle stick?
    a. check the patient's medical records
    b. decontaminate the site and fill out an incident report
    c. go to employee health service and get a tetanus booster
    d. leave the area so that the patient does not notice the injury

63. Which is *not* a symptom of shock?
    a. cold, clammy skin
    b. expressionless face and staring eyes
    c. increased shallow breathing
    d. strong, rapid pulse

64. The main principles involved in radiation exposure are:
    a. exposure time, amount of radiation, and glove thickness
    b. exposure time, distance, and shielding
    c. time of day, amount of radiation, and source
    d. time of day, distance, and eye protection

65. Infection control programs follow guidelines set by:
    a. College of American Pathologists
    b. Centers for Disease Control and Prevention
    c. Clinical Laboratory Improvement Amendments of 1988 (CLIA'88)
    d. NFPA

66. Which of the following is an example of a nosocomial infection? When a:
    a. catheter site of a patient in ICU becomes infected
    b. health care worker contracts hepatitis from a needlestick
    c. patient is admitted with Hanta virus
    d. pediatric patient breaks out with measles the day after admission for a tonsillectomy

67. Which organization's regulations supersede those of all other organizations?
    a. CAP
    b. CDC
    c. JCAHO
    d. OSHA

68. Which of the following contains regulations requiring availability of PPE in the medical laboratory?
    a. CLIA '88
    b. Food and Drug Agency Regulations
    c. Occupational Exposure to Blood-borne Pathogens Standard
    d. OSHA HAZCOM Standard

69. A patient who has a pathogenic organism transmitted by the fecal route would be in which type of isolation?

a. contact
b. enteric
c. respiratory
d. strict

70. The most prevalent infectious health hazard to a phlebotomist is:
a. HAV
b. HBV
c. HIV
d. TB

71. Which of the following is *not* a required part of an exposure control plan?
a. a body substance isolation statement
b. an exposure determination
c. communication of hazards
d. methods of implementation

72. Which class fire occurs with combustible metals?
a. A
b. B
c. C
d. D

73. Enteric isolation is used for patients with infections that are transmitted by:
a. droplets
b. fleas
c. ingestion
d. radiation

74. Which of the following is *not* an example of possible "parenteral" means of transmission?
a. drinking contaminated water
b. getting stuck by a needle used on a patient with AIDS
c. rubbing the eye with a contaminated hand
d. touching infectious material with chapped hands

75. Which of the following would *not* affect a person's general susceptibility to infection?
a. age
b. gender
c. health
d. immune status

76. An example of vector infection transmission is:
a. acquiring HIV infection from a blood transfusion
b. contracting hepatitis from a contaminated counter top
c. contracting plague from the bite of a rodent flea
d. TB transmitted by droplet nuclei

77. In what instance might a patient be placed in protective isolation? The patient has:
a. chicken pox
b. hepatitis
c. severe burns
d. tuberculosis

78. What is the correct order for removing protective clothing?
a. gloves, mask, gown
b. gown, gloves, mask
c. gown, mask, gloves
d. mask, gown, gloves

79. HBsAg is an indicator of:
a. HAV infection
b. HBV immunity
c. HBV infection
d. HIV infection

80. A radiation hazard symbol (Fig. 6-2) on a patient's door signifies a patient who:

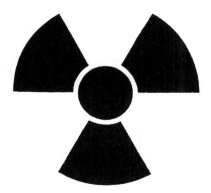

FIGURE 6-2. Radiation hazard symbol.

a. has gone to radiology
b. had many radiographs
c. is being treated with radioactive isotopes
d. needs to go to radiology

81. Which of the following is an example of a work practice control that reduces risk of exposure to blood-borne pathogens?
    a. a biohazard symbol
    b. an exposure control plan
    c. handwashing following glove removal
    d. HBV vaccination

82. Which institution introduced the concept of universal precautions?
    a. CAP
    b. CDC
    c. JCAHO
    d. OSHA

83. Health care workers are considered immune to a disease if they have:
    a. a normal white blood count
    b. had the disease
    c. received gamma globulin within the last year
    d. all the above

84. What should you use to extinguish a flammable liquid fire?
    a. class A extinguisher
    b. class B extinguisher
    c. fire blanket
    d. water

85. Which federal agency requires the labeling of hazardous materials?
    a. CDC
    b. JCAHO
    c. NFPA
    d. OSHA

86. Which type of contact infection transmission involves transfer of an infective microbe to the mucous membranes of a susceptible individual by means of a cough or sneeze?
    a. direct
    b. droplet

c. fomites
d. indirect

87. Which of the following is *not* a link (component) in the chain of infection?
    a. means of transmission
    b. source
    c. surveillance
    d. susceptible host

88. The organization specifically charged with the investigation and control of disease:
    a. CDC
    b. CLIA'88
    c. JCAHO
    d. OSHA

89. What is the proper order of first aid for shock?
    a. call for help, open airway, cover, elevate legs
    b. lower head, call for help, open airway, cover
    c. open airway, call for help, lower head, cover
    d. open airway, elevate legs, cover, give fluids

90. What is the first step to take if someone is choking and cannot talk or breathe?
    a. administer four backward chest thrusts
    b. call paramedics
    c. finger probe the throat
    d. give four quick blows to back

91. A nosocomial infection is:
    a. a laboratory acquired infection
    b. acquired by a patient while in the hospital
    c. always communicable
    d. detected by pre-admission screening tests

92. The type of transmission where the infection originated from contaminated food, water, drugs, or blood transfusion is:
    a. airborne
    b. contact

c. vector

d. vehicle

93. What procedure should be followed by a phlebotomist who has been diagnosed with strep throat?

   a. antibiotic therapy for 24 hours before returning to work

   b. evaluation by infection control personnel

   c. no special procedures if no symptoms are exhibited

   d. wear a mask when in contact with patients

94. Which of the following require an MSDS be supplied by the manufacturer?

   a. fluid-resistant laboratory coats

   b. most patient medications

   c. isopropyl alcohol

   d. isotonic saline

95. Which of the following is an example of an engineering control that helps eliminate hazards posed by blood-borne pathogens:

   a. gloves

   b. laboratory coat

   c. sharps container

   d. universal precautions statement

96. Manufacturers are required to supply MSDS for their products by:

   a. Blood-borne Pathogen Standard

   b. CDC regulations

   c. NFPA guidelines

   d. HAZCOM Standard

97. Infections that can be spread from person to person are called:

   a. communicable

   b. nonpathogenic

   c. nosocomial

   d. systemic

98. Which class of fire occurs with flammable liquids?

   a. class A

   b. class B

   c. class C

   d. class D

99. The first thing to do in the event of electrical shock to a co-worker or patient is:

   a. call for medical assistance

   b. keep the victim warm

   c. shut off the source of electricity

   d. start CPR

100. When a pathogen invades the body and causes disease the result is called a/an:

   a. chain of infection

   b. communicable disease

   c. infection

   d. systemic infection

ANSWERS TO REVIEW QUESTIONS

1. *d.* Typical proper nursery infection control techniques include wearing a mask, gown, and gloves because neonates in the ICU are more susceptible to infections than older children or adults.

2. *a.* The codeword or acronym established by the NFPA for the order of action steps in the event of fire is RACE and represents rescue, alarm, confine, and extinguish.

3. *d.* It is not mandatory for the source patient to submit to HIV or HBV testing

4. *c.* The process of infection requires the "chain of infection" to be complete. If the process is stopped or interrupted by such things as handwashing, the wearing of gloves, immunization, or instituting isolation procedures, infection will be prevented.

5. *d.* Universal precautions was introduced because it is not always possible to know if a patient is infected with a blood-borne pathogen.

6. *d.* Infection control programs follow regulations and guidelines established by OSHA, CDC, and JCAHO as well as other state and local regulatory agencies.

7. *c.* Not all facilities differentiate between respiratory isolation and AFB isolation. Because active tuberculosis can be transmitted through droplets (contact) or droplet nuclei all precautions are necessary, including wearing a mask, gloves, and gown.

8. *a.* Personal protective equipment, handwashing, and HBV vaccination are all recommended by OSHA's Blood-borne Pathogen Standard, but it is illegal to dismiss HIV-positive workers without just cause.

9. *c.* HIV is the leading cause of AIDS. HAV and HBV cause hepatitis A and hepatitis B, respectively.

10. *b.* Immunity to a particular antigen is said to exist when a person has antibodies to that antigen circulating in the blood. A person who has antigen remaining in the body but no longer displays symptoms of the virus is called a carrier. A person is infectious if he or she still carries the virus in his or her system. A person who is susceptible has little resistance to a disease.

11. *a.* Control of hemorrhage or abnormal bleeding is most effectively accomplished by elevating the affected part above the level of the heart and applying direct pressure to the wound.

12. *c.* An infection control program is responsible for implementing procedures designed to break the chain of infection and prevent the spread of infection in the hospital.

13. *b.* The majority of microscopic organisms (microbes) are nonpathogenic, meaning they do not cause disease under normal conditions. The microbes that are capable of causing disease are called pathogens.

14. *d.* TB is an infectious disease caused by the *Mycobacterium tuberculosis* organism. This organism is not normally present in the blood but is present in respiratory secretions and can be spread by droplet contact.

15. *d.* Clean paper towels should be used to turn off the faucet after handwashing because using the same paper towel that was used to dry the hands could contaminate the faucet handles.

16. *c.* Pertussis or whooping cough is a respiratory disease transmitted by airborne droplets. Chicken pox is highly contagious and requires strict isolation. Influenza requires contact isolation. *Shigella* is transmitted by ingestion and requires enteric isolation.

17. *b.* Class C fires occur with electrical equipment and require nonconducting agents to extinguish them.

18. *d.* Universal precautions should be followed at all times with no exceptions. All patients should be treated as if their blood and body fluids are infected with a blood-borne pathogen.

19. *a.* The procedure for HBV vaccination involves three separate injections: initial dose, another 1 month later, and another 6 months from the original injection.

20. *a.* Fomites are objects capable of adhering to infectious material and transmitting disease. Fomites can include telephones, computer terminals, and counter tops.

21. *c.* The OSHA HAZCOM Standard requires manufacturers of hazardous materials to supply MSDS for their products. An MSDS contains general, precautionary, and emergency information for the product. Because this information protects employees by ensuring that products will be used safely and for their intended purpose, the standard has become known as the "right to know" law.

22. *b.* Instructions for category-specific isolation are usually contained on a card placed on the patient's door.

23. *a.* Strict isolation, also called complete isolation, is required for patients with highly contagious diseases that can be spread by direct contact and through the air.

24. *c.* Hepatitis B virus (HBV) causes hepatitis as the name implies. The word hepatitis breaks down into the word root "hepat" which means liver and "itis" meaning inflammation.

25. *b.* Three components are necessary for a fire to occur. They are fuel, oxygen or an oxidizing agent, and heat for an ignition source.

26. *d.* The "chain of infection" can be broken or interrupted by such things as handwashing, the wearing of gloves, stress reduction, proper nutrition, and institution of isolation procedures.

27. *b.* All soiled articles should be placed in appropriate biohazard containers or bags according to the infection control system called *body substance isolation (BSI)*. Contaminated articles should never be thrown in the regular trash.

28. *d.* Electrical equipment should be unplugged before servicing to avoid electrical shock. Never handle electrical equipment with wet hands. Frayed electrical cords are dangerous. Extension cords should be avoided, if possible, because they lead to circuit overload as well as incomplete connections and potential clutter in the path of workers.

29. *d.* Before initiating CPR, responsiveness of the victim should be ascertained by gently shaking the victim and asking if he or she is okay.

30. *a.* Body substance isolation goes beyond universal precautions by requiring the wearing of gloves when contacting any body substance (Fig. 6-3).

31. *b.* A mask is necessary in respiratory isolation because of airborne transmission of the infective agent or droplet nuclei. Gloves are not always necessary but are required for phlebotomy procedures or other contact with blood and other body fluids.

32. *d.* Statistics compiled by the CDC have shown that needlesticks are responsible for approximately 50% of the HIV exposures that have occurred so far in the health care setting.

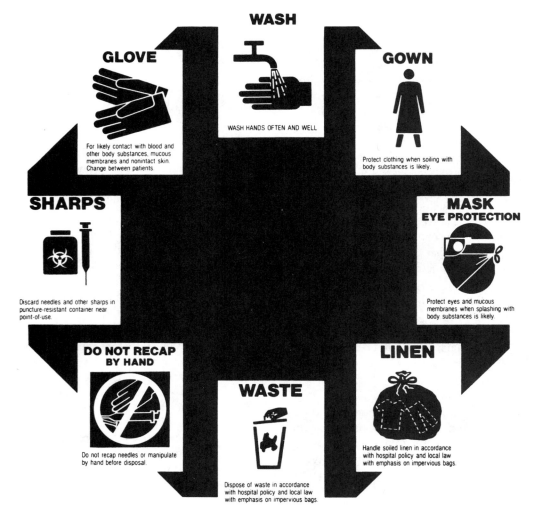

FIGURE 6-3. Body substance isolation sign. (Adapted from Briggs Corp., Des Moines, IA.)

33. *c.* The most common nosocomial infection in the United States is urinary tract infection (UTI). This condition could involve any of the organs and ducts participating in secretion and elimination of urine.

34. *d.* Health care employees face a serious health risk as a result of occupational exposure; consequently, OSHA put into force the Occupational Exposure to Blood-Borne Pathogens Standard. Enforcement of this standard is mandated by federal law.

35. *d.* A laboratory coat is considered PPE and as such may become contaminated with body fluids and blood; therefore, it should not be worn outside the laboratory during breaks or lunch. However, a separate clean laboratory coat may be worn at these times.

36. *b.* The phlebotomist should know the location of and how to use the safety eye wash station in the event of a chemical splash to the eye. Eyes should be flushed with water for a minimum of 15 minutes.

37. *b.* The proper way to remove a gown is from the inside by sliding the arms out of the sleeves and then folding it so that the contaminated outer surface is to the inside. It is left in a proper container in the room. All articles leaving the room must be double-bagged and labeled "biohazard" before disposal or decontamination for reuse.

38. *a.* The PPD test is a screening test for TB. All employees are required to be screened every 6 months.

39. *c.* Indirect contact involves the transfer of the pathogenic organism to the host through contact with contaminated articles of the infected person such as bed linens.

40. *a.* HBV, HIV, and the organism that causes syphilis are blood-borne pathogens and can be transmitted by transfusion if present in the transfused blood. Diabetes mellitus is a disorder of carbohydrate metabolism and results from inadequate production or use of insulin.

41. *d.* According to OSHA, gloves should be worn at all times when performing phlebotomy procedures. Protective isolation of HIV-positive patients and a mask worn by health care workers when treating these patients could occur should it become necessary for the patient's protection, but labeling the specimens as HIV-positive is not legal.

42. *d.* Figure 6-1 represents the NFPA "water reactive" symbol and is used to label hazardous chemicals that should not come in contact with water.

43. *b.* The word neutropenic means "a condition in which there is an abnormally low number of neutrophil cells in the blood." A neutrophil is a type of white blood cell. A patient with a low white blood cell count has increased susceptibility to infection. Therefore, neutropenic patients are sometimes placed in a type of protective or reverse isolation called "neutropenic" isolation.

44. *d.* To prevent contamination of other articles in the phlebotomist's tray or other workers who may handle it, a tube that has blood on it should be

wiped with disinfectant before being placed in the tray.

45. *a.* A stop sign (Fig. 6-4) requires anyone entering the room to check with the patient's nurse before entering. It is an alert to health care workers that precautions are to be followed when entering the room.

46. *a.* An employee with a positive PPD test would not have restrictions on working if results of chest radiographs were negative. An employee with influenza, rubella, or weeping dermatitis could spread the infection to others and would have work restrictions.

47. *c.* There are four classes of fire recognized by the NFPA. They are categorized by the fuel source of the fire.

48. *b.* Nosocomial infections can result from contact with infected personnel, other patients, visitors, or equipment. One of the best ways to prevent transmission of the pathogenic organism is proper handwashing.

49. *c.* Also called "reverse" isolation, this special kind of isolation is used for patients who are highly susceptible to infections. Examples of patients requiring protective isolation are neutropenic (low white blood count) and severely burned patients.

50. *a.* The word "percutaneous" is used to indicate direct inoculation through previously intact skin, such as that which occurs from accidental needlesticks and injuries from other sharp objects. Handling blood specimens with

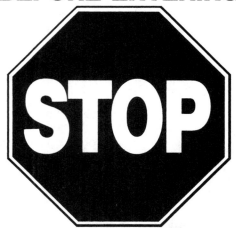

REPORT TO NURSE BEFORE ENTERING

STOP

FAVOR DE ANUNCIARSE A LA ENFERMERA DE PISO ANTES DE ENTRAR AL CUARTO

BRIGGS   L-9214   Des Moines, Iowa 50306   1-800-247-2343

FIGURE 6-4. Precaution "stop sign." (Adapted from Briggs Corp., Des Moines, IA.)

ungloved, chapped hands may cause contact transfer through the skin but is not considered inoculation. Mucous membrane contact with infectious material is called parenteral transmission.

51. *d.* Touching electrical equipment while drawing a patient's blood could cause a short to travel through the needle and shock the patient.

52. *c.* OSHA's HAZCOM Standard is also called the "right-to-know" law because all products with a hazardous warning on the label require an MSDS. This information helps ensure that products will be used safely and for their intended purpose.

53. *a.* Because not all types of isolation require the use of all PPEs, it is best to read the precaution signs on the patient's door. Stop signs on the doors of patients show the precautions to take or direct those who wish to enter the room to first check with the patient's nurse.

54. *c.* Blood-borne pathogen is a term applied to any infectious microorganism present in blood and other body fluids and tissues. It most commonly refers to HBV and HIV but also includes the organisms that cause syphilis, malaria, relapsing fever, and Creutzfeldt-Jakob disease. The organisms that cause influenza, rubella, and tuberculosis are not present in the blood.

55. *d.* Virulence deals with the degree to which the organism can cause the disease and how long between the time the source was contaminated and the host was contacted.

Viability is the ability of the organism to survive on the source. Susceptibility has to do with the immune system of the host and is affected by such things as age and health.

56. *a.* Biohazard is defined as anything that is harmful or potentially harmful to humans, other species, or the environment. "Bio" is a prefix indicating relationship to life. Biohazardous material is marked with a special symbol seen in Figure 6-5.

57. *c.* When putting on protective clothing, the health care worker puts on the gown first, being careful to touch only the inside surface. The mask is put on next. Gloves are applied last and pulled over the cuffs of the gown.

58. *b.* In the NFPA hazardous materials rating system the blue quadrant on the left indicates health hazard. The upper red quadrant indicates fire hazard. Stability or reactivity are indicated in the yellow quadrant on the right and a white quadrant on the bottom indicates other specific hazards (see Fig. 6-8).

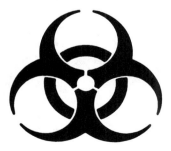

FIGURE 6-5. Biohazard symbol.

59. **b.** The Department of Transportation (DOT) labeling system (Fig. 6-6) uses a diamond-shaped warning sign incorporating the hazard symbol and number. This symbol should not be confused with the NFPA's diamond-shaped sign divided into four quadrants signifying specific hazards.

60. **c.** Mixing bleach with other cleaners can release dangerous gases.

61. **d.** An employee must be offered HBV vaccination within 10 days of employment in an area considered to have occupational exposure risk.

62. **b.** When an accidental needlestick occurs it is very important that the site be decontaminated immediately. The exposure should then be reported to the supervisor and an incident report filled out. The employee should also report to the employee health service for medical evaluation and possible treatment.

63. **d.** The symptoms of shock are pale, cold, clammy skin, shallow breathing rate, expressionless face, and weak (*not* strong), rapid pulse.

64. **b.** Distance, time, and shielding are the principles involved in radiation exposure and mean that the amount of radiation you are exposed to depends on how far you are from the source of radioactivity, how long you are exposed to it, and what protection you have from it.

65. **b.** The CDC, along with OSHA and JCAHO, establish guidelines for infection control programs.

66. **a.** A nosocomial infection is an infection that is acquired by a patient after admission to a health care facility. A catheter site that becomes infected while a patient is in the ICU is therefore a nosocomial infection. Infection of a health care worker is not considered a

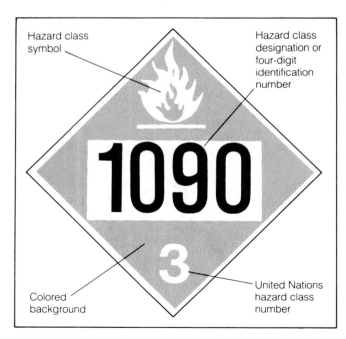

FIGURE 6-6. Example of DOT hazardous materials labels (flammable, poison, corrosive, etc.) (Jones SA, Weigel A, White RD, McSwain NE, Breiter M).

nosocomial infection. The patient admitted with Hanta virus obviously acquired the virus before admission. Because the incubation period for measles is longer than 1 day, the patient with measles acquired the infectious organism before being admitted to the hospital.

67. *d.* OSHA regulations, such as those concerning employee exposure to blood-borne pathogens, mandated by federal standard 1910.1030 are federal regulations or laws and therefore supersede all other organizations' requirements.

68. *c.* Availability of PPE in the laboratory is mandated by the OSHA Occupational Exposure to Blood-Borne Pathogens Standard to minimize occupational exposure to HBV, HIV, and other blood-borne pathogens.

69. *b.* A patient who has a pathogenic organism transmitted through feces would be confined to enteric isolation.

70. *b.* According to OSHA every year approximately 8700 health care workers contract hepatitis B and about 200 die as a result. This makes HBV the most frequently occurring laboratory-associated infection and a major infectious health hazard. HAV, HIV, and TB are also health hazards to health care workers, but they do not occur as frequently as HBV.

71. *a.* To comply with OSHA standards, an exposure control plan must contain a universal precautions statement, an exposure determination, communication of hazards, and methods of implementation.

72. *d.* Class D fires occur with combustible or reactive metals such as sodium, potassium, magnesium, and lithium.

73. *c.* The word "enteric" is defined as pertaining to the small intestine. Enteric isolation is used when the means of transmission is by ingestion.

74. *a.* Because the word "parenteral" means any route other than the digestive tract, all answers are examples of parenteral transmission except drinking contaminated water.

75. *b.* Gender does not play a role in a person's general susceptibility to infection. However, gender may play a role in the site of infection because of differences in male and female anatomy.

76. *c.* Vector transmission involves transfer of the microbe by an insect, arthropod, or animal, for example, the bite of a rodent flea.

77. *c.* Protective or reverse isolation is used for patients who are highly susceptible to infections as in the case with a severely burned patient.

78. *d.* The mask is removed first, being careful to touch only the strings. The gown is removed next, sliding the arms out of the sleeves and away from the body. It is folded with the outside (contaminated side) in. The gloves are removed last by grasping one glove at the wrist and pulling it inside out off the hand and holding it in the gloved hand. The second glove is removed by slipping the fingers under it at the wrist and pulling it inside out over the first glove so that the first glove ends up inside the second.

79. *c.* HBV infection is indicated by the presence of hepatitis B surface antigen (HBsAg) in the blood.

80. *c.* If the radiation hazard sign appears on a patient's door, it means the patient has been injected with radioactive dyes. Even in a patient, these radioactive isotopes can be hazardous to pregnant health care providers.

81. *c.* Work practice controls are routines that alter the manner in which a task is performed to reduce the likelihood of exposure, for example, handwashing following glove removal.

82. *b.* The CDC introduced this concept because it is not always possible to know if a patient is infected with a blood-borne pathogen.

83. *b.* Immunity to a particular disease is conferred by having had the disease and therefore developing antibodies against the disease-causing organism; or by vaccination against the particular organism. Gamma (immune) globulin confers temporary immunity. A normal white blood count is necessary to fight infection, but it is not an indication of immunity.

84. *b.* A flammable liquid or vapor fire requires blocking the source of oxygen or smothering the fuel to extinguish the fire. Class B or ABC extinguishers use dry chemicals to smother the fire.

85. *d.* OSHA's Hazardous Communication (HAZCOM) Standard requires labeling of hazardous materials and the labeling must comply with the requirements set by the Manufacturers Chemical Association.

86. *b.* Droplet contact transmission involves the transfer of infective organisms to the mucous membranes of the mouth, nose, or eyes of a susceptible individual by the sneezing, coughing, or talking of an infected person. The common cold is an example of infection that can be transmitted by droplets through coughing or sneezing.

87. *c.* A source of organisms, means of transmission of the organism, and the presence of a susceptible host are all "links" in the chain of infection. Surveillance is a means of monitoring and preventing infection or "breaking the chain of infection."

88. *a.* A division of the US Public Health Service called the Centers for Disease Control and Prevention (CDC) is charged with the investigation and control of various diseases, especially those that are communicable and have epidemic potential.

89. *c.* The proper order of first aid for shock is important and includes the following: opening the airway, calling for assistance, keeping the head lower than the rest of the body, and keeping the victim warm.

90. *a.* The first step is to administer four chest thrusts as in the Heimlich method.

91. *b.* Approximately 5% of patients in the United States contract (acquire) some sort of infection after admission to a health care facility. Such infections are called nosocomial infections.

92. *d.* Vehicle transmission involves the transmission of an infective microbe through contaminated food, water, drugs, or blood products. Shigella

infection from contaminated water and hepatitis infection from blood products are examples of vehicle transmission.

93. *a.* A phlebotomist diagnosed with strep throat is not allowed to work until he or she has been on antibiotic therapy for a minimum of 24 hours and is not exhibiting symptoms. Once allowed to return to work, a mask is not necessary and neither is an evaluation by infection control personnel.

94. *c.* Any product that has a hazardous warning on the label must have an MSDS supplied by the manufacturer. Isopropyl alcohol has a hazardous warning on the label, therefore an MSDS is required. Laboratory coats, saline, and most patient medications do not have hazard warnings and do not require an MSDS.

95. *c.* An engineering control is an item or device, such as a sharps container, eyewash station, or self-sheathing needle, that isolates or removes the hazard from the work place.

96. *d.* The HAZCOM Standard from OSHA requires manufacturers to supply MSDS for their products. These sheets contain general information as well as precautionary and emergency information for the product.

97. *a.* Diseases that can spread from person to person are called "communicable infections."

98. *b.* Class B fires occur with flammable liquids and vapors such as paint, oil, grease, or gasoline.

99. *c.* A person's first reaction during the event of an electrical shock is to try to remove the person from the source of the electricity, but this can result in shock to the rescuer if the source of electricity is still there. The first thing to do, therefore, is to shut off the source of electricity.

100. *c.* If a pathogen invades the body and the conditions are favorable for it to multiply and cause injurious effects or disease, the resulting condition is called an infection.

Blood Collection Equipment and Supplies

7

A. **General Blood-Drawing Equipment**
   1. *Blood-Drawing Station*
   2. *Carts and Trays*
   3. *Gloves*
   4. *Antiseptics and Disinfectants*
   5. *Sterile Gauze Pads*
   6. *Bandages*
   7. *Needles and Sharps Disposal Containers*
   8. *Slides*
B. **Venipuncture Equipment**
   1. *Tourniquets*
   2. *Needles*
   3. *Evacuated Tube System*
      a. *Components of the System*
         (1) *Holders*
         (2) *Evacuated Tubes*
      b. *Tube Additives*
         (1) *Anticoagulants*
         (2) *Antiglycolytic Agent*
         (3) *Clot Activators*
         (4) *Thixotropic Gel Separator*
      c. *Tube Stoppers*
   4. *Order of Draw*
      a. *Evacuated Tube Method*
      b. *Syringe Method*
         (1) *Syringe System*
         (2) *Winged Infusion Set*

REVIEW QUESTIONS

1. Which is the *best* tube for collecting an ethanol specimen?
   a. ethylenediaminetetraacetate (EDTA)
   b. siliceous earth
   c. sodium citrate
   d. sodium fluoride

2. Which type of anticoagulant is normally used to collect a specimen for a complete blood count (CBC)?
   a. EDTA
   b. heparin
   c. sodium citrate
   d. no anticoagulant is needed

3. Which is *not* true of disinfectants? Disinfectants are:
   a. corrosive chemical compounds
   b. safe to use on human skin
   c. used to kill pathogenic microorganisms
   d. used on surfaces and instruments

4. Which needle gauge has the largest bore?
   a. 18
   b. 20

c. 21
d. 22

5. Which of the following procedures is *most* likely to increase the chance of hemolyzing a specimen? Using a:
   a. 21-gauge needle and evacuated tube system to collect a specimen from the median cubital vein
   b. 22-gauge needle and syringe to collect a specimen from a difficult vein
   c. 23-gauge butterfly needle to collect a specimen from a hand vein
   d. 25-gauge butterfly needle to collect a specimen from a child

6. What department would use a sodium polyanetholesulfonate (SPS) tube?
   a. chemistry
   b. coagulation
   c. hematology
   d. microbiology

7. Blood collected in a red stopper tube:
   a. may be used for most coagulation tests
   b. will not clot
   c. yields plasma and cells
   d. yields serum and clotted red cells

8. This test is collected in a light-blue stopper tube.
   a. glucose
   b. platelet count
   c. prothrombin time (PTT)
   d. red blood cell count

9. A green stopper tube normally contains:
   a. EDTA
   b. heparin
   c. lithium
   d. sodium citrate

10. Which of the following is a required characteristic of a sharps container?
    a. bright red or orange in color
    b. leak-proof and puncture-resistant
    c. marked with a biohazard symbol
    d. all of the above

11. What is the purpose of the rubber sleeve that covers the tube end of a multiple-sample needle?
    a. enables smooth tube placement and removal
    b. maintains sterility of the sample
    c. prevents leakage of blood during tube changes
    d. protects the needle and keeps it sharp

12. The *best* solution to use to clean up blood is:
    a. alcohol
    b. povidone iodine
    c. soap and water
    d. sodium hypochlorite

13. The part of the evacuated tube holder that is meant to aid in smooth tube removal:
    a. barrel
    b. flange
    c. hub
    d. sleeve

14. All of the following additives interfere with the action of calcium in the clotting process except:
    a. EDTA
    b. heparin
    c. potassium oxalate
    d. sodium citrate

15. Which of the following tubes are in the proper order of draw for the syringe method?
    a. lavender, light blue, red
    b. light blue, lavender, red
    c. light blue, red, lavender
    d. red, lavender, light blue

16. The purpose of sodium citrate in specimen collection is:
    a. accelerates clotting
    b. inhibits glycolysis
    c. preserves glucose
    d. protects coagulation factors

17. Which of the following stopper colors designates a tube used for coagulation testing?

a. green
b. lavender
c. light blue
d. red

18. Which size needles are used for routine venipuncture?
    a. 16–18 gauge
    b. 18–20 gauge
    c. 20–22 gauge
    d. 22–24 gauge

19. What does the "gauge" of a needle refer to?
    a. diameter
    b. length
    c. strength
    d. volume

20. What is the purpose of an antiglycolytic agent?
    a. enhances clotting
    b. inhibits electrolyte breakdown
    c. preserves glucose
    d. prevents clotting

21. Why are gauze pads rather than cotton balls considered a better choice for covering the site while holding pressure following venipuncture?
    a. gauze pads are more sterile
    b. gauze pads create more pressure
    c. cotton balls are not as absorbent
    d. cotton fibers tend to stick to the site

22. Which of the following substances is contained in a serum separator tube?
    a. EDTA
    b. heparin
    c. sodium citrate
    d. thixotropic gel

23. Mixing equipment from different manufacturers can result in:
    a. improper needle fit
    b. needle coming unscrewed
    c. tubes popping off
    d. all of the above

24. A royal-blue top tube with a green label contains:
    a. EDTA
    b. heparin
    c. no additive
    d. sodium citrate

25. Solution used to clean the site before routine venipuncture:
    a. 5.25% sodium hypochlorite
    b. 70% isopropyl alcohol
    c. 70% methanol
    d. povidone iodine

26. When disposable latex tourniquets (Fig. 7-1) become soiled with blood, it is best to:
    a. autoclave them before reuse
    b. throw them away

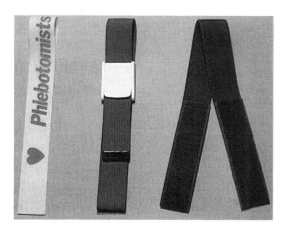

FIGURE 7-1. *Several types of tourniquets (left to right): latex strap, Seraket®, and velcro closure.*

c. wash them in bleach

d. wipe them with alcohol

27. What is the *most* important factor in choosing which gauge needle to use for venipuncture?

    a. age of the patient

    b. number of tubes to be collected

    c. size and condition of the patient's vein

    d. type of test being collected

28. Which additive is usually present in a lavender stopper tube?

    a. acid citrate dextrose

    b. citrate

    c. EDTA

    d. heparin

29. This tube stopper indicates that the tube contains sodium citrate:

    a. green

    b. lavender

    c. light blue

    d. royal blue

30. In which instance is needle recapping recommended?

    a. after collecting a specimen in a syringe

    b. after collecting a specimen in the emergency room

    c. after collecting blood gases

    d. recapping is *never* a recommended procedure

31. The *best* choice of equipment for drawing difficult veins is:

    a. butterfly and evacuated tube holder

    b. lancet and Microtainer®

    c. needle and evacuated tube holder

    d. needle and syringe

32. Glass particles present in serum separator tubes:

    a. accelerate coagulation

    b. deter clotting

    c. inhibit glycolysis

    d. prevent hemolysis

33. Evacuated tubes are coated with silicon to:

    a. allow the tubes to fill more quickly

    b. keep red blood cells from clinging to the tube

c. prevent glycolysis

d. prevent reflux of tube contents

34. Which of the following can be used as a clot activator?

    a. EDTA

    b. heparin

    c. silica

    d. thixotropic gel

35. Heparin prevents blood from clotting by:

    a. activating calcium

    b. binding calcium

    c. heparin does not prevent clotting

    d. inhibiting thrombin

36. The part of the syringe measured in cc or mL is called the:

    a. adapter

    b. barrel

    c. hub

    d. plunger

37. Which of the following should *not* be used on infants under 2 years of age?

    a. adhesive bandages

    b. evacuated tubes

    c. isopropyl alcohol

    d. tourniquet

38. Which of the following is normally used to clean the site when collecting blood culture specimens?

    a. benzalkonium chloride

    b. isopropanol

    c. povidone iodine

    d. sodium hypochlorite

39. The slanted tip of the needle that enters the vein is called the:

    a. bevel

    b. gauge

    c. hub

    d. lumen

40. Which anticoagulant is contained in a serum separator tube?

    a. EDTA

    b. heparin

    c. no anticoagulant

    d. sodium citrate

41. Which tube is filled last when using a syringe?
    a. EDTA
    b. heparin
    c. nonadditive
    d. sterile

42. When collecting specimens for a CBC, PTT, and blood urea nitrogen (BUN) what is the proper order of draw using the evacuated tube method?
    a. lavender stopper, light-blue stopper, red stopper
    b. light-blue stopper, lavender stopper, red stopper
    c. red stopper, lavender stopper, light-blue stopper
    d. red stopper, light-blue stopper, lavender stopper

43. A "STAT" test that is often collected in a lithium heparin containing tube is:
    a. blood cultures
    b. CBC
    c. electrolytes
    d. PTT

44. Which of the following prevents the metabolism of glucose?
    a. EDTA
    b. heparin
    c. silica
    d. sodium fluoride

45. Which of the following needle gauges has the smallest diameter?
    a. 18
    b. 21
    c. 22
    d. 23

ANSWERS TO REVIEW QUESTIONS

1. *d.* A gray stopper tube containing potassium oxalate and sodium fluoride prevents coagulation and glycolysis and is used for alcohol determinations as well as glucose tests. Alcohol values are stable because glycolysis is prevented.

2. *a.* EDTA is the anticoagulant of choice for whole blood hematology studies because it preserves blood cell morphology and prohibits platelet aggregation.

3. *b.* Disinfectants are corrosive chemical compounds that are bactericidal (kill bacteria). Some also kill viruses, such as human immunodeficiency virus (HIV) and hepatitis. Disinfectants are used on surfaces and instruments to kill potential pathogens. They are *not* safe for use on human skin.

4. *a.* The needle gauge with the largest bore or lumen is the one with the smallest number.

5. *d.* A 25-gauge butterfly needle is sometimes successfully used to collect blood specimens on infants and others with difficult veins, but any time a needle smaller than 23 gauges is used to collect blood the chance of trauma to the red blood cells and resulting hemolysis is increased.

6. *d.* The tube containing SPS is used in the collection of blood cultures which are performed in the microbiology department. SPS is an anticoagulant with special properties that prevents phagocytosis of bacteria.

7. *d.* Blood collected in tubes without additives, for example, red stopper or gold stopper serum separator tubes, will clot and yield serum on centrifugation. Most coagulation tests are performed on plasma, *not* serum. Anticoagulated specimens yield plasma and cells when centrifuged.

8. *b.* A PTT is a coagulation test and is collected in a light-blue stopper containing sodium citrate. A platelet count is sometimes ordered to assess coagulation, but is a hematology test collected in a lavender stopper.

9. *b.* Green stopper tubes contain one of three heparin formulations: ammonium, lithium, or sodium heparin.

10. *d.* The Occupational Safety and Health Administration (OSHA) requires that sharps containers (Fig. 7-2) be bright red or orange, marked with a biohazard label, leak-proof, rigid, puncture-resistant, disposable, easily sealed when full, and contain a device to aid in needle removal.

11. *c.* The rubber sleeve of a multiple sample needle retracts as the needle is inserted into the tube, allowing the tube to fill with blood, and recovers the needle as the tube is removed, preventing leakage of blood into the tube holder.

12. *d.* A 1:10 dilution of household bleach (5.25% sodium hypochlorite) is recommended for cleaning blood spills because it has been shown to be effective at killing hepatitis B virus (HBV) and (HIV).

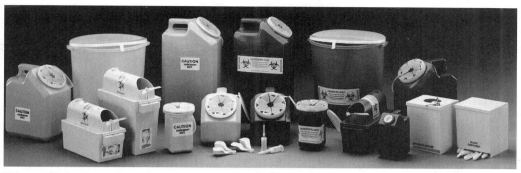

Figure 7–2 Several styles of sharps containers. (Courtesy of PRO TEC Containers, Inc., Irvine, CA)

13. *b.* The flanges or extensions on the sides of the tube end of the holder are there to aid in tube placement and removal.

14. *b.* Calcium is essential to the coagulation process. EDTA, sodium citrate, and potassium oxalate bind or precipitate calcium, making it unavailable to the coagulation process. Heparin prevents coagulation by inhibiting the clotting component thrombin.

15. *b.* With the exception of sterile specimens that are collected first in either method, the order of filling evacuated tubes with blood obtained by syringe differs from the evacuated tube order of draw. It is assumed that the blood that enters the syringe last is the freshest and will be the first blood out of the syringe in the transfer process. Because the clotting process has already been activated as the blood fills the syringe, it is important to fill the tubes that require anticoagulants first. Of the anticoagulant tubes, the light blue is the most critical because it is affected most by activation of the coagulation process. EDTA tubes are filled next because microclot formation causes erroneous hematology test results. Serum tubes are filled last because they are supposed to clot.

16. *d.* Sodium citrate protects the coagulation factors and is used in light-blue stopper tubes for coagulation testing.

17. *c.* The light-blue stopper tube contains sodium citrate as the additive. Sodium citrate prevents coagulation by binding calcium and is the anticoagulant of choice for coagulation studies performed on plasma.

18. *c.* Evacuated tube system needles are available in 20- to 22-gauge sizes, with 21-gauge needles most commonly used for routine venipuncture.

19. *a.* The gauge of the needle indicates the size of the needle and refers to the diameter of the lumen or internal space of the needle.

20. *c.* An antiglycolytic agent is a substance that inhibits glycolysis (metabolism of glucose) by the cells of the blood.

21. *d.* Fibers from cotton or rayon balls tend to stick to the site and reinitiate bleeding when removed.

22. *d.* Thixotropic gel is an inert (nonreacting) synthetic substance that forms a physical barrier between the cellular portion of a specimen and the serum or plasma portion after the specimen has been centrifuged. When used in a serum collection tube it is called serum separator. When used in a plasma collection tube it is called plasma separator.

23. *d.* Although evacuated tube collection system components from different manufacturers are similar, they are not necessarily interchangeable. Mixing components from different manufacturers can lead to problems, such as needles coming unscrewed or tubes popping off during venipuncture procedures.

24. *b.* The royal-blue stopper tube may contain either sodium heparin, sodium EDTA, or no additive. The label is color coded red, green, or lavender, indicating which additive is present. The royal-blue stopper color indicates that the tube and stopper offers the lowest verified levels of trace elements available.

25. *b.* The most common antiseptic used for routine blood collection is 70% isopropyl alcohol (isopropanol). A 5.25% sodium hypochlorite solution (bleach) is a disinfectant and is not safe to use on human skin. Povidone iodine is used for collection of sterile specimens such as blood cultures. Methanol can be toxic when absorbed through the skin and is not used as a skin antiseptic.

26. *b.* The most commonly used tourniquet is a flat strip of stretchable latex. A soiled latex tourniquet can easily be wiped clean with disinfectant. However, if soiled with blood, the bleach required to kill blood-borne pathogens disintegrates latex and makes it gummy. Because latex tourniquets are relatively inexpensive, they are usually discarded if soiled with blood.

27. *c.* The age of the patient, number of tubes to be collected, and the type of test being collected all play a part in equipment selection for venipuncture, but ultimately, it is the size and condition of the patient's vein that dictates what equipment, including needle gauge, is selected.

28. *c.* Lavender stopper tubes contain EDTA which is the anticoagulant of choice for whole blood hematology studies. EDTA prevents coagulation by binding calcium in the form of a potassium or sodium salt.

29. *c.* A light blue stopper indicates that the tube contains sodium citrate. A royal-blue stopper sometimes contains EDTA, but only if it has a lavender label. A royal-blue stopper indicates that the tube and stopper are as free of trace elements as possible. A green stopper indicates a heparin-containing tube and a light-blue stopper indicates the presence of sodium citrate unless it has a special yellow.

30. *d.* Used needles must be disposed of immediately in special containers

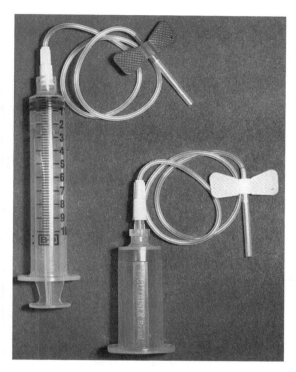

FIGURE 7-3. Winged infusion sets: *(left)* attached to a syringe; *(right)* attached to evacuated tube holder by means of a luer adapter.

usually referred to as "sharps" containers. Needles *must not* be recapped, cut, bent, or broken before disposal.

31. *a.* A winged infusion set or butterfly needle (Fig. 7-3) is an indispensable tool for collecting blood from small or difficult veins because it allows much more flexibility and precision than either a regular needle and evacuated tube holder or needle and syringe. A lancet and microtainer can be used for some specimens, but there are a number of tests that cannot be collected by skin puncture.

32. *a.* Glass particles present in serum separator tubes provide increased surface for platelet activation consequently increasing or accelerating the speed of clotting.

33. *b.* Some evacuated tubes, especially those for serum determinations, are coated on the inside with silicon to help prevent destruction of red blood cells and to keep the blood from sticking to the sides of the tube.

34. *c.* A clot activator is a substance that initiates or enhances coagulation. Clot activators include substances that provide increased surface for platelet activation, such as glass or silica particles and inert clays like siliceous earth and celite, as well as the clotting components thromboplastin and thrombin.

35. *d.* Heparin prevents coagulation by inhibiting the clotting component thrombin. Thrombin is necessary for the formation of fibrin from fibrinogen. Without thrombin, a fibrin clot cannot form.

36. *b.* The barrel of a syringe holds the fluid being aspirated and is measured in cc or mL. The hub is where the needle attaches. The plunger fits within the barrel. Pulling on the plunger creates the vacuum that fills the syringe (Fig. 7-4).

37. *a.* Adhesive bandages should not be used on infants under 2 years of age because of the danger of aspiration and suffocation.

38. *c.* Povidone iodine, often referred to by the trade name Betadine, is the recommended antiseptic for cleaning blood culture collection sites.

39. *a.* The end of the needle that is inserted into the vein is called the bevel (see Fig. 7-4) because it is cut on a slant or "beveled" to allow the needle to penetrate the vein easily and prevent coring (removal of a portion of the

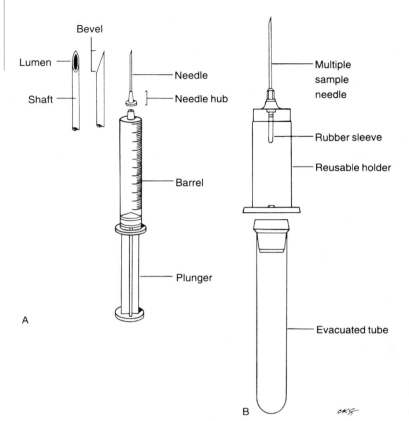

FIGURE 7-4. **(A)** Syringe components; **(B)** Components of the evacuated tube collection system.

skin or vein). The gauge of a needle refers to the internal diameter. The hub of a needle is the end that attaches to a syringe or tube holder. The lumen of a needle is the internal space of the needle.

40. *c.* There is no anticoagulant in a serum separator tube. A serum separator tube contains silica to enhance coagulation and an inert gel that forms a physical barrier between the serum and the cells after centrifugation.

41. *c.* Blood that enters the syringe first is the oldest and will be the last blood out of the syringe in the transfer process; therefore, it

should be put in nonadditive tubes which will clot.

42. *d.* The proper order of draw using the evacuated tube method is red, light blue, and lavender. When multiple tubes are to be drawn, an order of draw is recommended to avoid contamination of nonadditive tubes by additive tubes, as well as cross-contamination between different types of additive tubes.

43. *c.* Electrolytes are chemistry tests traditionally performed on serum, but to save the time it takes for a serum specimen to clot before it can be tested, "STAT" electrolytes and other "STAT" chemistry tests are

often performed on plasma specimens collected in heparin tubes.

44. *d.* Metabolism of glucose is called glycolysis. A substance that prevents glycolysis is called an antiglycolytic agent. The most common antiglycolytic agents are sodium fluoride and iodoacetic acid.

45. *d.* The larger the gauge number, the smaller the actual diameter of the needle. Of the gauges listed, a 23-gauge needle would have the smallest diameter.

Factors to Consider Prior to Blood Collection

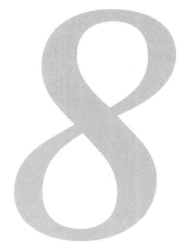

A. **Physiological Factors**
1. Basal State
2. Factors Influencing Basal State
   a. Age
   b. Altitude
   c. Dehydration
   d. Diurnal Variations
   e. Diet
   f. Drugs
   g. Environment
   h. Exercise
   i. Position
   j. Pregnancy
   k. Gender
   l. Stress

B. **Test Status**
1. STAT
2. Medical Emergency
3. Timed Specimens
4. ASAP
5. Fasting
6. Pre-op
7. Routine
8. Routine Admission

C. **Factors to Consider in Site Selection**
1. Scars and Burns
2. Mastectomy
3. Hematoma
4. Edema
5. Obesity
6. Damaged Veins
7. Intravenous Therapy
8. Vascular Access Devices

   a. Central Venous Catheter
     (1) Broviac
     (2) Groshong
     (3) Hickman
   b. Arterial Line
9. Heparin Lock
10. Cannula
11. Fistula

D. **Complications Associated With Blood Collection**
1. Complications Affecting the Patient
   a. Allergies to Antiseptics and Adhesives
   b. Seizures
   c. Excessive Bleeding
   d. Fainting
   e. Hematoma
   f. Infection
   g. Nausea
   h. Pain
   i. Petechiae
   j. Reflux of Anticoagulant
   k. Vein Collapse
   l. Vein Damage
   m. Nerve Damage
   n. Inadvertent Arterial Puncture
2. Collection Techniques Affecting Specimen Integrity
   a. Hemoconcentration/Venous Stasis
   b. Hemolysis
   c. Partially Filled Tubes
   d. Specimen Contamination

REVIEW QUESTIONS

1. An indwelling line consisting of tubing that has been surgically inserted into a main vein or artery is called a/an:
   a. cannula
   b. fistula
   c. heparin lock
   d. VAD

2. Persistent diarrhea in the absence of fluid replacement may cause:
   a. hemoconcentration of the blood
   b. hemolysis of red blood cells
   c. high white blood cell count
   d. low iron (Fe) levels

3. What physical changes occur when a patient goes from supine to standing?
   a. calcium levels decrease
   b. nonfilterable blood elements increase
   c. plasma volume increases
   d. RBC counts decrease

4. The phlebotomist must collect a specimen on a patient in the intensive care unit (ICU). The patient has difficult veins and the nurse has agreed to draw the specimen from an arterial line if the phlebotomist assists with the collection. What is the proper procedure for drawing an ammonia, complete blood count (CBC), and protime from an arterial line using the evacuated tube system?
   a. clear the line and draw a green, lavender, and blue top tube
   b. draw the blue immediately, then lavender and green
   c. draw a 10-mL discard tube, then blue, green, and lavender
   d. draw a 5-mL discard tube followed by blue, lavender, and green

5. What tests may be affected most if the patient is not fasting?
   a. blood culture and thyroid profile
   b. CBC and protime
   c. glucose and triglycerides
   d. rheumatoid arthritis (RA) and cardiac enzymes

6. A specimen that is ordered STAT should be collected:
   a. as soon as possible
   b. immediately
   c. on the next scheduled sweep
   d. within 1 hour

7. The phlebotomist must collect a STAT hemoglobin from an ICU patient. There is an intravenous (IV) catheter in the left arm. There is no suitable antecubital vein or hand vein in the right arm. What should the phlebotomist do?
   a. call another phlebotomist to draw the specimen
   b. collect the specimen by skin puncture
   c. draw a hand vein below the IV
   d. draw the specimen from an ankle vein

8. Which of the following is most affected by altitude?
   a. bilirubin
   b. electrolytes
   c. glucose
   d. red blood cell count

9. Which vein is often the one most easily palpated on obese patients?
   a. basilic
   b. brachial
   c. cephalic
   d. median cubital

10. The following tests have all been ordered at the same time on different inpatients. There is only one phlebotomist on duty. Which test should the phlebotomist collect first?
    a. ASAP CBC in oncology
    b. hemoglobin in labor and delivery
    c. timed blood cultures in ICU
    d. STAT electrolytes in the emergency room (ER)

11. Which of the following need *not* be avoided when choosing a venipuncture site?

a. edematous areas
b. damaged veins
c. petechiae
d. scars and burns

12. The ratio of anticoagulant to blood is most critical for which of the following tests?
    a. bilirubin
    b. CBC
    c. electrolytes
    d. prothrombin time

13. When a blood specimen is drawn from a heparin lock, which of the following procedures should be followed? Draw:
    a. a 5-mL discard tube before the test specimen
    b. an extra tube for each test
    c. coagulation specimens first
    d. more blood than needed for the test

14. Which of the following tests requires the patient's age when calculating results?
    a. CPK
    b. creatinine clearance
    c. human immunodeficiency virus (HIV)
    d. glucose

15. Which instance most closely resembles basal state? A patient who has:
    a. been lying down for an hour
    b. just arrived for a fasting blood test
    c. just awakened at 0600 after fasting since the evening meal last night
    d. worked all night but was fasting all night at work

16. You must draw a protime from a patient with IVs in both arms. Which of the following is the best thing to do? Draw the specimen:
    a. above the IV
    b. below the IV
    c. from an ankle vein
    d. from the IV

17. Which of the following factors known to affect basal state is automatically accounted for when establishing reference values for tests?
    a. diurnal variations
    b. effects of interfering drugs
    c. exercise effects
    d. geographic environmental factors

18. According to the College of American Pathologists, drugs known to interfere with urine tests should be discontinued how many hours before the test?
    a. 4–24
    b. 12–24
    c. 24–36
    d. 48–72

19. Which is the best way to avoid reflux?
    a. don't release the tourniquet until the last tube
    b. draw while the patient is in a supine position
    c. keep the patient's arm straight
    d. make certain the tubes fill from the bottom up

20. Which of the following is least likely to cause hemolysis of a specimen?
    a. collecting more than one tube of blood
    b. mixing tubes too vigorously
    c. pulling blood into a syringe too quickly
    d. using a needle with too small a bore

21. A vein that feels cord-like and lacks resilience may be:
    a. an artery
    b. collapsed
    c. superficial
    d. thrombosed

22. It is not a good idea to collect a CBC specimen from a screaming infant because the:
    a. platelets are more likely to clump
    b. specimen will be hemoconcentrated
    c. specimen will be more likely to hemolyze
    d. white blood count may be falsely elevated

23. Medical emergency (Med Emerg) means the same as:
    a. ASAP
    b. pre-op
    c. routine
    d. STAT

24. Which of the following is least likely to result in hematoma formation when collecting a specimen by venipuncture?
    a. inadequate pressure is applied to the site after needle withdrawal
    b. the needle has penetrated through the back of the vein
    c. the needle bevel is centered in the lumen of the vein
    d. the needle bevel is only partly inserted in the vein

25. You have no choice but to draw a specimen from a site with a hematoma. Where should you obtain the specimen?
    a. distal to the hematoma
    b. in the area of the hematoma
    c. proximal to the hematoma
    d. none of the above

26. Which of the following tests is *most* likely to be ordered STAT?
    a. bilirubin
    b. electrolytes
    c. erythrocyte sedimentation rate
    d. glucose tolerance test

27. Central venous catheters (CVCs) include all of the following except:
    a. Broviac
    b. Groshong
    c. Heparin lock
    d. Hickman

28. Which laboratory test has higher reference values for males than for females?
    a. cholesterol
    b. glucose
    c. HCT
    d. potassium

29. The serum or plasma of a lipemic specimen would appear:
    a. cloudy
    b. dark yellow
    c. foamy
    d. pink to red

30. Which liquid is acceptable to drink when fasting?
    a. black coffee
    b. milk
    c. tea
    d. water

31. Prolonged tourniquet application may cause a change in blood composition primarily because of:
    a. hemoconcentration
    b. hemoglobin
    c. hemolysis
    d. homeostasis

32. The serum or plasma of a hemolyzed specimen would appear:
    a. clear yellow
    b. cloudy
    c. dark yellow
    d. pink or reddish

33. Which of the following situations is *least* likely to cause contamination of the specimen?
    a. collecting an ethanol specimen after cleaning the site with isopropyl alcohol
    b. drawing a blood culture specimen before the povidone iodine has dried
    c. cleansing the site with alcohol before collecting a PKU specimen
    d. using povidone iodine to clean a skin puncture site

34. Allow alcohol to dry before venipuncture to avoid:
    a. a stinging sensation
    b. hemoconcentration
    c. hemostasis
    d. petechiae

35. Drawing blood from an edematous extremity may cause:
    a. erroneous results
    b. hemolysis of the specimen

c. premature clotting of the specimen
d. none of the above

36. Why should scarred or burned areas be avoided as blood collection sites?
   a. newly burned sites may be painful and are susceptible to infection
   b. scarred sites may have impaired circulation and yield erroneous results
   c. veins are difficult to palpate in such areas
   d. all of the above

37. Which of the following is affected most by muscular activity?
   a. bilirubin
   b. calcium
   c. enzymes
   d. glucose

38. Routine admission tests are tests that are:
   a. commonly ordered by physicians to establish a diagnosis or monitor a patient's progress
   b. required of all patients by the health care facility
   c. required before surgery
   d. used in therapeutic drug monitoring

39. Breakage or rupture of red blood cells is called:
   a. hematocrit
   b. hemoconcentration
   c. hemolysis
   d. hemostasis

40. A phlebotomist has attempted twice to draw a partial thromboplastin time on a patient with difficult veins. Both times the phlebotomist has been able to draw only a partial tube. What should the phlebotomist do?
   a. collect the specimen by skin puncture
   b. have another phlebotomist attempt to draw the specimen
   c. pour the two tubes together and mix well
   d. send the tube with the most blood to the laboratory with a note that it was a difficult draw

41. Which is *not* a reason to control temperature and humidity in a laboratory?
   a. because reference values are established under controlled conditions
   b. to insure proper functioning of equipment
   c. to lessen drug interference
   d. so that specimen integrity is maintained

42. A lipemic specimen is a clue that the patient was:
   a. dehydrated
   b. fasting
   c. in a basal state
   d. not fasting

43. Why do pregnant patients have lower reference ranges for red blood cell counts?
   a. body fluid increases in pregnancy have a diluting effect on red blood cells
   b. constant nausea leads to hemoconcentration of red blood cells
   c. poor appetite leads to transient anemia
   d. the growing fetus uses up the mother's iron reserves

44. The *best* specimen for use in establishing inpatient reference ranges is a:
   a. basal state specimen
   b. fasting specimen
   c. steady-state specimen
   d. two-hour post prandial specimen

45. Excessive or blind probing for a vein can cause:
   a. diurnal variation
   b. lipemia
   c. nerve damage
   d. petechiae

46. An abnormal accumulation of fluid in the tissues that causes swelling is called:
   a. a hematoma
   b. edema
   c. hemolysis
   d. thrombosis

47. Which of the following tests is most often a timed test?
    a. blood urea nitrogen
    b. complete blood count
    c. therapeutic drug monitoring
    d. rapid plasma reagin

48. An outpatient faints while a blood specimen is being collected. What should the phlebotomist do?
    a. lower the patient's head and continue to draw the specimen
    b. remove the needle from the patient's arm and lower the patient's head and arms
    c. remove the needle from the patient's arm and shake the patient to bring him or her to consciousness
    d. use one hand to hold the patient upright and continue to draw the specimen

49. Erroneous laboratory results can be caused by:
    a. hemoconcentration
    b. hemolysis
    c. lipemia
    d. all of the above

50. The most common complication from a venipuncture is:
    a. hematoma
    b. petechiae
    c. seizures
    d. syncope

51. An outpatient becomes weak and pale following a blood collection procedure. What should the phlebotomist do?
    a. have someone accompany the patient to his or her car
    b. have the patient lie down
    c. offer the patient a drink of water
    d. tell the patient to go get something to eat right away

52. This blood component exhibits diurnal variation with peak levels occurring in the morning.
    a. bilirubin
    b. calcium
    c. cortisol
    d. glucose

53. Which instance may lead you to suspect that you have accidentally punctured an artery?
    a. a hematoma starts to form instantly
    b. the blood obtained is dark red in color
    c. the blood pulses into the tube
    d. there is no way to tell

54. A pre-op patient:
    a. has just been admitted to the hospital
    b. has just had an operation
    c. is an outpatient
    d. is going to have surgery

55. If blood is drawn too quickly from a small vein, the vein will have a tendency to:
    a. bruise
    b. collapse
    c. disintegrate
    d. roll

56. How long before obtaining blood for testing should drugs known to interfere with blood tests be discontinued:
    a. 1 to 4 hours
    b. 4 to 24 hours
    c. 24 to 36 hours
    d. 48 to 72 hours

57. Avoid drawing blood from an arm on the same side as a mastectomy because the
    a. arm is usually edematous
    b. effects of lymphostasis may yield erroneous results
    c. veins in that arm will more easily collapse
    d. none of the above

58. A fistula is a/an:
    a. implanted port attached to an indwelling line
    b. permanent fusion of an artery and a vein

c. special winged infusion set left in a patient's arm

d. temporary fusion of an artery and a vein

59. Small red spots that appear after a tourniquet is applied are called:
    a. capillaries
    b. hematomas
    c. petechiae
    d. thrombi

60. Which of the following is *not* likely to impair vein patency?
    a. improperly redirecting the needle
    b. leaving the tourniquet on for 2 minutes
    c. numerous venipunctures in the same area
    d. probing for a deep vein

ANSWERS TO REVIEW QUESTIONS

1. *d.* An indwelling line surgically inserted into a main vein or artery is called a vascular access device (VAD). A cannula is a temporary surgical connection between an artery and a vein. A fistula is a permanent surgical fusion of an artery and a vein. A heparin lock is a special winged needle set inserted into a vein.

2. *a.* Hemoconcentration is a condition in which some blood components, such as red blood cells, enzymes, and electrolytes may be falsely elevated because of a decrease in total body fluid noticeably changing the ratio of analytes in the plasma.

3. *b.* When a patient stands up after being supine (lying down), the plasma of the blood filters into the tissues causing a decrease in plasma volume and an increase in nonfilterable elements of the blood such as calcium and red blood cells.

4. *c.* The order of draw from an arterial line using the evacuated tube system is the same as a regular evacuated tube system draw. However, a discard tube is required before collecting the specimens because the lines are routinely flushed with heparin. A 10-mL discard tube is required for coagulation tests. A 5-mL discard tube is all that is needed for other tests.

5. *c.* Glucose levels will be elevated if the patient has eaten recently and can even be affected by chewing gum and drinking black coffee. Triglycerides appear in the bloodstream after ingestion of fatty foods and may stay elevated for up to 12 hours. Results of the other tests listed are not affected by diet.

6. *b.* Stat comes from the Latin word "statim," and means immediately. Stat requests should not only be drawn immediately, but also should be processed and results reported immediately.

7. *b.* The most expedient thing to do in this situation is to collect the hemoglobin by skin puncture. A skin puncture specimen could be collected and on its way to the laboratory in the time it would take for another phlebotomist to come to draw the specimen, the IV to be shut off for 2 minutes so that the specimen could be collected below it, or permission obtained to draw from an ankle vein.

8. *d.* The red blood cell count is most affected by a change in altitude because the decrease in oxygen content of the air at higher altitudes causes the body to produce more red blood cells to fulfill the body's oxygen requirements.

9. *c.* The cephalic vein is often the one most easily palpated on obese patients.

10. *d.* Certain test requests take precedence over others, and with only one phlebotomist on duty, it is important to assess each test request and determine the order of priority. Of the tests listed, STAT electrolytes in the ER should be collected first because of the critical values that can occur with potassium levels. A CBC in oncology to be collected as soon as possible (ASAP) does not take priority over a STAT in ER. A hemoglobin in labor and delivery is important but can wait because it had no priority attached to the order. A blood culture that is not collected on time may result in delay

of treatment to the patient but is not life threatening.

11. *c.* Scars and burns, edematous areas, and damaged veins should all be avoided when choosing a venipuncture site. Petechiae are caused by the application of the tourniquet and may not be avoidable because they will probably occur at any site that is chosen. The presence of petechiae will not compromise test results.

12. *d.* A prothrombin test is a coagulation test. The ratio of anticoagulant to blood is most critical for coagulation tests because a ratio of one part anticoagulant to nine parts of blood must be maintained for accurate results. The excess anticoagulant in a short draw will dilute the plasma portion of the specimen on which the test is performed and falsely prolong results.

13. *a.* When blood is drawn from a heparin lock, a 5-mL discard tube must be drawn first to eliminate residual heparin used to flush the lock and keep it from clotting. Drawing coagulation specimens from a heparin lock is not recommended.

14. *b.* Some physiologic functions, such as clearance of creatinine by the kidneys, decrease with age, and results are calculated using the patient's age as well as body surface.

15. *c.* A patient who has just awakened at 0600 and has not eaten since about 1800 the night before is said to be in "basal state" meaning the patient has been resting and fasting for approximately 12 hours before the blood is drawn.

16. *b.* According to the National Committee for Clinical Laboratory Standards, a specimen can be drawn below an IV after the nurse shuts the IV off for a minimum of 2 minutes. The fact that the IV was turned off should be indicated on the requisition form along with the initials of the nurse. Never draw a specimen from above an IV as the specimen may be contaminated with fluid from the IV. Only specially trained personnel may draw specimens from IVs. Drawing coagulation specimens from ankle veins is not recommended. In addition collecting specimens from ankle veins can only be done with the physician's permission.

17. *d.* Reference values for tests are established using basal state specimens. Environmental factors associated with geographic location will affect basal state. However, because all the specimens used to calculate reference values come from patients in that particular location, the geographical factors will be the same for all the specimens and will automatically be reflected in the results.

18. *d.* According to the College of American Pathologists (CAP), drugs known to interfere with urine testing should be avoided for 48 to 72 hours before urine sample collection.

19. *d.* Reflux can occur when the blood in the tube is in contact with the needle. This can be prevented by keeping the arm downward during blood collection so that the tube fills from the bottom up.

20. *a.* Mixing tubes too vigorously, pulling blood into a syringe too quickly, and using too small of a needle can all result in hemolysis of the specimen. Blood collection systems are designed to collect multiple tubes of blood

without affecting the specimen in any way.

21. **d.** A vein that is thrombosed feels hard, cord-like, and lacks resilience. A superficial vein will have resilience; an artery will pulsate; and a collapsed vein cannot be palpated.

22. **d.** A white blood cell count is part of a CBC. Studies performed on crying infants demonstrated marked increases in white blood cell counts. These increases were temporary and returned to normal once the infant had been calm for approximately 1 hour. Therefore, collecting a CBC specimen from a crying infant may result in a falsely elevated white blood cell count.

23. **d.** Some institutions have started using the designation "Med Emerg" in place of "STAT" to identify specimens that are needed to respond to critical situations.

24. **c.** Hematoma formation can be caused by many different errors in technique.

The needle centered in the lumen of the vein is exactly where the needle should be and will cause no problems.

25. **a.** When drawing from an area with a hematoma it is best to go below (distal) to the hematoma where the blood flow is not affected by the presence of the hematoma.

26. **b.** Abnormal electrolyte balance can be life-threatening and requires immediate corrective action. Therefore, electrolytes are often ordered "STAT."

27. **c.** A CVC (Fig. 8-1) is an indwelling line inserted into a main vein such as the subclavian and advanced into the vena cava. Broviac, Groshong, and Hickman are all types of CVCs. A heparin lock is a device inserted into a patient's vein to allow access for administering medications.

28. **c.** A patient's gender has a determining effect on the concentration of

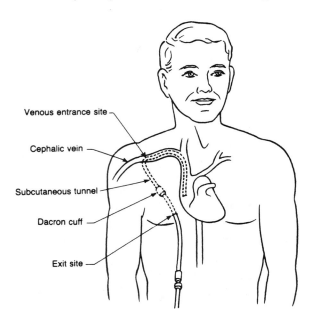

Venous entrance site
Cephalic vein
Subcutaneous tunnel
Dacron cuff
Exit site

FIGURE 8-1. Central venous catheter (CVC) (Metheny NM).

numerous blood components including hematocrit (HCT). These differences are reflected in separate normals for males and females.

29. *a.* Serum or plasma that has fatty substances (lipids) dissolved in it appears cloudy or turbid. The term used to describe this condition is *lipemia*, and the term used to describe how the serum looks is *lipemic*.

30. *d.* The only liquid acceptable to drink when fasting is water.

31. *a.* Prolonged tourniquet application causes stagnation of the blood flow (venous stasis). This causes the plasma portion of the blood to filter into the tissues resulting in an increase in nonfilterable blood components or hemoconcentration.

32. *d.* Hemolysis is the destruction of red blood cells and the liberation of hemoglobin into the serum or plasma portion of the specimen. This causes the serum or plasma to appear pink or reddish depending on the degree of hemolysis and the specimen is described as being "hemolyzed."

33. *c.* Cleaning the site with alcohol before PKU collection is proper technique. Using isopropyl alcohol to clean the site before blood alcohol (ethanol) collection will invalidate the results. Povidone iodine residue can inhibit microorganism growth in blood cultures leading to false-negative results. Povidone iodine should not be used to clean skin puncture sites because it interferes with the following tests: bilirubin, uric acid, phosphorous, and potassium (BURPP).

34. *a.* Performing venipuncture before the alcohol has dried may cause a stinging sensation to the patient. It may also cause slight hemolysis of the specimen.

35. *a.* Edema impairs circulation and may disrupt exchange of oxygen and nutrients between the blood and tissues. Test results of specimens collected from edematous areas would therefore be erroneous.

36. *d.* Scarred and burned areas should be avoided as blood collection sites because they can be painful, can yield erroneous results, and can be difficult to palpate.

37. *c.* Muscular activity will elevate the blood levels of a number of blood components including enzymes. After exercise, creatine phosphokinase and lactate dehydrogenase may remain elevated 24 hours or more.

38. *b.* Routine admission tests are those tests commonly required of all patients by the health care facility.

39. *c.* Breakage or lysis of red blood cells is called hemolysis. (See answer to question 32.)

40. *b.* Partially filled coagulation tubes are unacceptable for testing. Pouring two partially filled tubes together would cause an improper ratio of blood to anticoagulant and is unacceptable. A partial thromboplastin time (PTT) cannot be collected by skin puncture. A phlebotomist should never make more than two attempts at venipuncture on a patient at one time. Therefore the best answer is to have another phlebotomist attempt to draw the specimen.

41. *c.* Temperature and humidity are known to affect test values; therefore, these environmental factors are closely controlled in the laboratory to insure specimen integrity as well as proper functioning of equipment. These environmental factors have no effect on drug interference.

42. *d.* A lipemic (cloudy) specimen signals that the patient may not be fasting. The ingestion of fatty substances causes triglycerides to be evident in the blood because they are being transported as lipoproteins and are insoluble in water.

43. *a.* Normal body fluid increases in pregnancy have a diluting effect on red blood cells, therefore reference ranges for red blood cell counts are lower. Reference ranges are established using specimens from normal pregnant women. Anemia from poor appetite or inadequate iron reserves represent situations that may result in values for the patient that are lower than the normal reference ranges. Hemoconcentration would most likely elevate red blood counts.

44. *a.* Reference ranges for laboratory tests on hospital patients (inpatients) are usually established using basal state specimens.

45. *c.* Excessive or blind probing for a vein can lead to injury of a main nerve, such as the median cutaneous nerve, causing permanent damage and the possibility of a lawsuit.

46. *b.* Accumulation of fluid in the tissues that causes the area to look swollen is called edema. It is often caused by infiltration of fluid from an IV line. Edema can also be caused by congestive heart failure.

47. *c.* Therapeutic drug monitoring is performed at timed intervals to determine peak and trough levels of the drug in the patient's system so that drug therapy is maximized. The other tests are not normally timed tests.

48. *b.* If an outpatient faints during venipuncture, immediately remove the needle from the patient's arm and lower his or her head. Stay with the patient until he or she is fully recovered to avoid injury to the patient and possible liability issues.

49. *d.* Hemoconcentration can cause an increase in nonfilterable blood components. Hemolysis, depending on the severity, can affect tests such as potassium and enzymes. Lipemia causes turbidity in the sample which may interfere with the testing process.

50. *a.* All of the choices are possible complications of venipuncture, but hematoma formation is the most common. Petechiae are only seen if the patient has platelet or vascular integrity problems. Seizures and syncope (fainting) are sometimes brought on by the stress of the blood draw.

51. *b.* An outpatient who becomes weak and pale after blood collection should be encouraged to lie down until he or she recovers. Offer the patient some juice and crackers once he or she recovers. The patient should not drive for at least 30 minutes.

52. *c.* Diurnal variation or normal fluctuation throughout the day is exhibited by the analyte cortisol with the highest levels occurring in the morning.

53. *c.* Blood pulsing or spurting into the tube is an indication that you may have punctured an artery.

54. *d.* "Pre-op" means before an operation and indicates the patient is on the way to surgery.

55. *b.* Drawing blood too quickly from a small vein may cause the vein to collapse. This is temporary and may occur when using a tube that is too large for the size of the vein or from pulling the plunger back too quickly when using a syringe.

56. *b.* Drugs known to interfere with blood tests should be avoided for 4 to 24 hours before testing according to the College of American Pathologists.

57. *b.* After a mastectomy or the removal of a breast, a patient's physician may request that blood not be drawn from the arm on the same side for a long period of time. Specimens collected from that arm may yield erroneous results as a result of lymphostasis caused by lymph node removal. These patients are also more susceptible to infection.

58. *b.* A fistula is a permanent surgical fusion of an artery and a vein. It is most commonly used for dialysis purposes and should not be used for collecting blood specimens.

59. *c.* Small, nonraised red spots that appear when a tourniquet is applied are called petechiae. They may be caused by defective capillary walls or platelets. They are an indication that the site may bleed excessively following venipuncture.

60. *b.* Leaving the tourniquet on for 2 minutes is not likely to impair vein patency or state of being freely open. It may, however, lead to erroneous results caused by hemoconcentration. Probing, improperly redirecting the needle, and numerous venipunctures in the same area are all actions that may impair the patency of a vein.

Venipuncture Collection Procedure

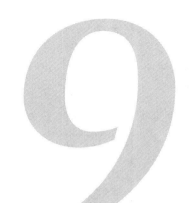

A. Initiation of the Test Request
1. Test Requisitions
2. Information Needed on the Requisition
3. Receipt of Test Requisition by the Laboratory
4. Preparing to Collect Requested Specimen

B. Patient Contact
1. Entering Patient Room
2. Identifying Yourself
3. Handling Special Situations
   a. Sleeping Patient
   b. Unconscious Patient
   c. Physician or Clergy With Patient
   d. Patient Not in Room
4. Handling Family and Visitors

C. Patient Identification
1. Importance
2. Patient Name and Date of Birth
3. Checking Identification Bracelet
4. Handling Discrepancies
5. Missing Identification
6. Emergency Room Identification
7. Infants and Young Children
8. Outpatients

D. Preparing the Patient for Testing
1. Bedside Manner
2. Handling Difficult Patients
3. Explaining the Procedure
4. Handling Patient Inquiries
5. Handling Patient Objections
6. Verifying Diet Restrictions

E. Routine Venipuncture Steps
1. Prepare Paperwork
2. Identify Patient
3. Verify Diet Restrictions
4. Assemble Equipment and Supplies
5. Put on Gloves
6. Reassure Patient
7. Position Patient
   a. Seated
   b. Supine
   c. Other Considerations
8. Apply Tourniquet
9. Select Site
10. Release Tourniquet
11. Verify Tube Selection
12. Cleanse Site
13. Reapply Tourniquet
14. Position Equipment and Remove Needle Sheath
15. Anchor Vein
16. Insert Needle
17. Fill Tubes
18. Release Tourniquet
19. Withdraw Needle
20. Dispose of Needle
21. Label Tubes
22. Observe Special Handling Instructions
23. Check Patient's Arm and Apply Bandage
24. Dispose of Contaminated Materials
25. Thank the Patient
26. Remove Gloves and Wash Hands
27. Check Specimen Collection Logs
28. Transport the Specimen to Laboratory

F. Failure to Obtain Blood
1. Tube Position and Vacuum
2. Needle Position

REVIEW QUESTIONS

1. You are about to draw blood from a patient. You touch the needle to the skin, but change your mind and pull the needle away. What do you do next?
   a. clean the site and try again using the same needle
   b. immediately try again using the same needle
   c. obtain a new needle before trying the procedure again
   d. wipe the needle across the alcohol pad and try again

2. Which of the following is *not* part of informed consent as related to the phlebotomist?
   a. advising the patient of his or her prognosis
   b. informing the patient that you are a student
   c. telling the patient that you will be drawing a blood specimen
   d. telling the patient the name of the test ordered

3. You have a request to draw a specimen on an inpatient by the name of John Doe. How do you proceed to identify (ID) your patient once you have identified yourself?
   a. ask the patient "Are you Mr. John Doe?"
   b. ask the patient to please state his name
   c. check the patient's ID band and say "I see that you are John Doe."
   d. if the ID band and requisition match, draw the specimen

4. It is acceptable to use an ankle vein when:
   a. coagulation tests are ordered
   b. the patient is paralyzed
   c. there is no other suitable site
   d. you have the physician's permission

5. Using information from the computer requisition (Fig. 9-1) identify the number that signifies the accession number:

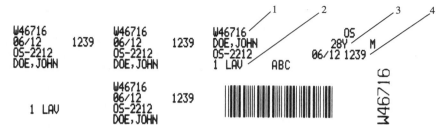

FIGURE 9-1. Computer requisition (Sunquest System, courtesy J. C. Lincoln Hospital, Phoenix, AZ.)

a. 1
b. 2
c. 3
d. 4

6. Using information from the computer requisition (see Fig. 9-1) identify the number that signifies the type of tube to be drawn:
a. 1
b. 2
c. 3
d. 4

7. What happens if you put pressure on the gauze while the needle is being removed?
a. it is painful
b. it prolongs needle removal
c. the needle may slit the skin
d. all of the above

8. Which of the following *should not* be used to enhance the vein selection process?
a. have the patient vigorously pump his fist
b. lower the arm
c. palpate the antecubital area
d. use a warm towel to increase blood flow

9. Which is *not* proper technique for collecting specimen tubes when using the evacuated tube method?
a. fill each tube until the vacuum is exhausted.
b. collect a "clear" tube before a coagulation tube.

c. collect nonadditive tubes before additive tubes
d. allow the tube to fill from the stopper end first

10. Which is the proper way to anchor a vein?
a. anchoring is not necessary
b. pull the skin taut with your thumb
c. use your index finger above and thumb below the site
d. none of the above

11. Using information from the computer requisition (see Fig. 9-1) identify the number that signifies the time ordered:
a. 1
b. 2
c. 3
d. 4

12. Which of the following information on a requisition must match information on the patient's ID band?
a. medical record number
b. physician
c. room number
d. test status

13. What is the best angle to use for needle insertion?
a. less than 15 degrees
b. 15 to 30 degrees
c. 30 to 45 degrees
d. angle does not matter

14. Before obtaining a blood specimen from a child, you must do all of the following *except*:
    a. establish rapport with the child and parent
    b. greet parent and child
    c. tell the child it won't hurt
    d. tell the child what to expect

15. Your patient is not wearing an ID band. You see that the ID band is taped to the night stand. The information matches your requisition. What do you do?
    a. ask the patient to state his or her name and go ahead and draw the specimen if the name matches
    b. ask the patient's nurse to attach an ID band before you draw the specimen
    c. fill out an incident form and return to the laboratory without drawing the specimen
    d. go to the nurses station. Make out an ID for the patient. Attach it and proceed to draw the specimen

16. Dorsal hand vein procedure on infants involves all of the following *except:*
    a. applying a latex tourniquet
    b. cleansing the area with isopropyl alcohol
    c. identifying the patient
    d. inserting the needle in a superficial vein

17. What should you do if the needle remains in the removal slot instead of dropping all the way into the sharps container during disposal?
    a. carefully lift it by the rubber sleeve and drop it into the container
    b. leave it alone, it will drop in eventually
    c. shake the sharps container until the needle drops in
    d. use the tube holder to carefully slide it to the wider end of the removal slot

18. You arrive to draw a fasting specimen. The patient is just finishing a big breakfast. What do you do?
    a. check with the patient's nurse first; if the specimen is collected, write "nonfasting" on the laboratory slip
    b. collect the specimen anyway because he or she just finished eating
    c. collect the specimen but write "nonfasting" on the laboratory slip
    d. refuse to collect the specimen and fill out an incident report slip

19. What is the National Committee for Clinical Laboratory Standards (NCCLS) recommended way to clean a venipuncture site?
    a. any way; just scrub as vigorously as you can
    b. wipe in ever-increasing concentric circles starting in the center
    c. wipe using concentric circles from the outside in
    d. all of the above

20. What do you do if the patient's physician is in the room and the specimen is ordered STAT?
    a. ask the patient's nurse what to do
    b. come back later when the physician has gone
    c. explain why you are there and ask permission to proceed
    d. excuse yourself and proceed to collect the specimen

21. What may happen if you mix tubes too vigorously?
    a. hemoconcentration
    b. hemolysis
    c. lipemia
    d. vigorous mixing has no affect

22. Proper immobilization of the pediatric patient for venipuncture involves all of the following *except:*
    a. a pair of phlebotomists, an immobilizer, and a blood drawer
    b. allowing the child to sit alone with his one arm bracing the other

   c. cradling the child close to the immobilizer

   d. phlebotomist grasping the child's wrist in a palm up position

23. How can you tell when the needle is in the vein as you insert it into the patient's arm?
   a. the needle will start to vibrate
   b. you will feel a slight "give"
   c. you will hear a hissing sound
   d. there is no way to tell

24. Your patient is cranky and rude to you. What do you do?
   a. ask the patient's nurse to draw the specimen
   b. be as polite and professional as you can and draw the specimen in your normal way
   c. do not speak to the patient; just get the necessary blood work and leave
   d. refuse to draw the patient's blood and leave

25. Never leave a tourniquet on for more than:
   a. 30 seconds
   b. 45 seconds
   c. 1 minutes
   d. 3 minutes

26. What precautionary information should you give an outpatient before you let him or her leave following venipuncture?
   a. advise him or her not to carry a bag or purse on that arm
   b. caution him or her not to lift heavy objects for at least 1 hour
   c. tell him or her to leave the bandage on for a minimum of 15 minutes
   d. all of the above

27. How can you tell that you are in a vein when using a needle and syringe?
   a. the blood will pump into the syringe if you are in a vein
   b. there is no way to tell
   c. you cannot tell until you pull back on the plunger and see blood
   d. you should see blood appear in the hub of the needle

28. When is the best time to release the tourniquet during venipuncture?
   a. as soon as blood flows freely into the tube
   b. as soon as the needle penetrates the skin
   c. after the last tube is collected
   d. after the needle is withdrawn

29. Which of the following situations is *least* likely to cause a vein to collapse?
   a. multiple tubes are being collected
   b. too large a tube is being used to collect the specimen for the size of the vein
   c. the patient is elderly and has "fragile" veins
   d. the plunger of a syringe is pulled too quickly while extracting the blood

30. What is the most critical error a phlebotomist can make
   a. collecting a timed specimen late
   b. failing to obtain a specimen from a patient
   c. giving a patient a hematoma
   d. misidentifying a patient specimen

31. It is important to fill anticoagulant tubes until the vacuum is exhausted in order to ensure that:
   a. the specimen clots properly
   b. there is a proper ratio of blood to anticoagulant
   c. there is adequate volume of blood to perform the test
   d. tissue fluid contamination of the specimen is minimized

32. More blood can be obtained on neonates with minimal trauma by using a:
   a. lancet on the great toe
   b. pediatric lancet on the heel
   c. small gauge needle in a dorsal hand vein
   d. syringe and butterfly in an antecubital vein

33. How often do you mix nonadditive tubes?
   a. 1 or 2 inversions
   b. 3 to 5 inversions

c. 5 to 10 inversions

d. nonadditive tubes do not require mixing

34. The *best* way to collect a PKU specimen from a dorsal hand vein is:
    a. allow the blood to drip into an EDTA microcollection tube
    b. collect the blood with a syringe
    c. let the blood drip onto the PKU card
    d. all of the above

35. How many times should most anticoagulant tubes be mixed?
    a. 2 or 3 inversions
    b. 5 to 10 inversions
    c. 10 to 12 inversions
    d. additive tubes do not require mixing

36. What would be the system of choice to identify laboratory specimens from an unconscious, unidentified woman in the emergency room?
    a. assign a name to the patient such as Jane Doe
    b. assign a number to the patient until admitted
    c. use a three-part identification band and labels
    d. wait to process specimens until the patient can be identified

37. Your inpatient is asleep when you arrive to draw blood, what do you do?
    a. check the ID and draw him or her quickly before he or she wakes up
    b. come back later when the patient is awake
    c. fill out a form that says you were unable to obtain the specimen because the patient was asleep
    d. shake the bed gently and call out the name softly

38. What is the proper arm position for venipuncture?
    a. in a downward position, but bent at the elbow
    b. straight from shoulder to wrist and in a downward position with the palm up

c. straight from shoulder to wrist with the palm down

d. the position of the arm doesn't matter

39. What may happen if the arm is bent up at the elbow to apply pressure after the venipuncture?
    a. bleeding may occur when the arm is lowered
    b. bruising may occur
    c. the platelets may pull away when the arm is straightened
    d. all of the above

40. You are in the process of collecting a blood specimen. Blood flow has been established. As the tube is filling you hear a hissing sound and there is a spurt of blood into the tube and the flow then stops. What has most likely happened is the:
    a. needle bevel came partly out of the skin and the vacuum escaped from the tube
    b. needle went through the vein
    c. patient's blood pressure dropped
    d. tube had a crack in it and there was no more vacuum

41. Success of blood collection for pediatric patients is most dependent on:
    a. aseptic technique
    b. order of draw
    c. patient immobilization
    d. tourniquet application

42. Proper identification of a patient *does not* include:
    a. asking the patient to state or spell his or her name
    b. comparing information on the requisition to the ID band
    c. match tube information to the ID and the requisition
    d. saying to the patient "Are you Mr. Jones?" etc.

43. What happens if you advance the tube past the guideline on the holder before needle insertion?

a. the tube will fail to fill with blood
b. the vacuum will be lost
c. you will have to get a new tube
d. all of the above

44. Which of the following is *not* mandatory information for the specimen label?
a. first and last name
b. hospital number or date of birth
c. phlebotomist's initials
d. room number and bed

45. Which instance would be proper identification of an outpatient?
a. asking the patient to state or spell his name
c. checking the patient's identification bracelet
c. verifying identification by a name tag from the patient's place of employment
d. writing the patient's name on the specimen label

46. Why is a patient's identification number included on the specimen tube label?
a. for insurance identification and payment purposes
b. so that it can be used for an accession number in the laboratory
c. to avoid confusing multiple specimens from the same patient
d. to avoid confusing specimens from patients with the same name

47. What is the advantage of using a butterfly?
a. blood flow is increased
b. butterflies are less expensive
c. butterflies make it easier to draw difficult veins
d. there is a greater choice of needle sizes

48. What does a sclerosed vein feel like?
a. hard and cord-like
b. it pulsates
c. resilient
d. soft and mushy

49. It is important for the phlebotomist to visually inspect the needle tip before inserting it in a patient's vein to:

a. check for the presence of bacteria
b. ensure that the bevel is down during insertion
c. make certain that the needle is not outdated
d. see if the needle point has imperfections that might damage the patient's vein

50. Before a specimen can be collected, the phlebotomist must *first* ensure that the:
a. laboratory performs the test
b. patient is in a basal state
c. patient's physician has been notified
d. the test request has been authorized

51. You are in the middle of drawing a blood specimen using the evacuated tube method. You realize that you filled the EDTA tube before the green stopper. What can you do?
a. draw the green one next and hope that there is no carryover
b. draw several milliliters into a plain discard tube; then fill the green one
c. it is acceptable to draw the EDTA before the green stopper
d. skip the green tube and come back later to collect it

52. Why should you remove the evacuated tube from the needle before withdrawing it from the patient's arm?
a. to be able to mix the tube as soon as possible
b. to decrease the pain felt by the patient on withdrawal
c. to prevent blood from dripping out of the needle after withdrawal
d. to reduce the chance of reflux

53. A butterfly and 23-g needle is the *best* choice to use on children less than 2 years old because:
a. children like the idea of the butterfly
b. children's veins are often sclerotic
c. flexibility of tubing allows for the child's movement
d. it eliminates excessive bleeding tendencies

54. Routine inpatient blood specimens should be labeled:
    a. at the bedside immediately after collection
    b. before the specimen is collected
    c. in the laboratory after collection
    d. outside the patient's room

55. Where is the tourniquet applied?
    a. 3 to 4 inches above the venipuncture site
    b. directly above the venipuncture site
    c. distal to the venipuncture site
    d. 10 inches above the venipuncture site

56. What happens if the tourniquet is too tight?
    a. arterial flow may be stopped
    b. hemoconcentration
    c. it hurts the patient
    d. all of the above

57. What is the most important step in specimen collection?
    a. patient identification
    b. proper specimen handling
    c. selecting the correct specimen tube
    d. tourniquet application

58. After penetrating a hand vein with a butterfly, the phlebotomist needs to "seat" the needle, meaning:
    a. have the patient make a tight fist to keep the needle in place
    b. keep the skin taut during the entire process
    c. slightly thread the needle up the central area of the vein
    d. push the needle up against the back wall of the vein

59. You arrive to draw a specimen on an inpatient. The patient's door is closed. What do you do?
    a. knock softly and open the door slowly, checking to see if it is all right to enter
    b. knock softly and wait for someone to come to the door
    c. leave to draw another patient and come back later
    d. open the door and proceed into the room

60. It is important to mix anticoagulant tubes immediately after filling them in order to:
    a. encourage coagulation
    b. inhibit hemoconcentration
    c. minimize hemolysis
    d. prevent microclot formation

61. When drawing blood from an older child the most important consideration is:
    a. explaining the importance of holding still
    b. explaining the tests that are being ordered
    c. giving the child some type of reward
    d. stating the reason for the test

62. You must collect a specimen on a 6 year old. The child is a little fearful. What do you do?
    a. explain what you are going to do in simple terms and ask the child for cooperation
    b. have someone restrain the child and go ahead and draw the specimen without explanation
    c. tell the child not to worry because it won't hurt
    d. tell the child that you will give him or her a treat if he or she doesn't cry

63. A patient vehemently refuses to allow you to collect a blood specimen. What should you do?
    a. convince the patient to cooperate
    b. have the nurse physically restrain the patient and proceed to collect the specimen
    c. notify the patient's nurse and fill out a "failure to collect specimen" form
    d. return to the laboratory and cancel the request

64. Use several thicknesses of gauze during needle removal so that:
    a. blood won't contaminate your glove
    b. it won't hurt when you pull the needle out

c. the patient doesn't see you pull the needle out

d. the site will stop bleeding sooner

65. When must you wash your hands when performing a routine blood draw?
    a. after glove removal
    b. before and after the blood draw
    c. before approaching the patient
    d. washing hands is not necessary if you wear gloves

66. When transferring blood from a syringe to evacuated tubes, which is the proper technique?
    a. force the blood in the tubes by pushing the syringe plunger
    b. hold the tube steady while penetrating the stopper
    c. place the evacuated tube in a rack before penetrating stopper
    d. none of the above

67. Which of the following should *not* be a cause of inability to obtain blood? The:
    a. needle has penetrated all the way through the vein
    b. needle is centered in the lumen of the vein
    c. needle is only partially inserted into the vein
    d. tube has lost its vacuum

68. The patient asks if the test you are about to draw is for diabetes. How do you answer?
    a. If the test is for glucose, say "yes it is."
    b. say that you don't know
    c. tell the patient that it is not, even if it is
    d. tell the patient that it's best to discuss the test with his or her physician

69. Why is it better to use gauze and not cotton balls for pressure over the site? Cotton balls:
    a. are less sterile
    b. may irritate the patient's skin
    c. may pull the platelets away when removed
    d. soak up too little blood

70. An unconscious patient does not have an ID band. The name and room number on the door agree with the requisition. What should you do?
    a. call your supervisor and ask what to do
    b. do not draw the patient until the nurse has applied an ID bracelet
    c. draw the blood and fill out an incident report form
    d. draw the patient and then ask the nurse to identify him or her

71. You are in the process of drawing a blood specimen from a patient in the ER. As you withdraw the needle from the patient's arm you discover that someone has moved your blood drawing tray and you can no longer reach the sharps container. What is the *best* action to take?
    a. hand the needle to the closest person and ask him or her to dispose of it for you
    b. hold the needle as high in the air as you can until you are finished holding pressure on the site
    c. stick the needle in the bed until you are finished with the patient
    d. use a one-handed procedure to resheath the needle temporarily until you can access your tray

72. You are in the process of collecting a specimen. The needle is inserted but the blood is filling the tube very slowly. You see a hematoma forming very rapidly. What has most likely happened is the:
    a. needle is only partly inserted in the vein
    b. needle is up against the vein wall
    c. patient has a coagulation problem
    d. tube is loosing vacuum

73. Which is *not* an acceptable reason for failure to obtain a blood specimen?
    a. the patient refused
    b. the patient was not available

    c. you attempted but were unable to obtain the blood

    d. you didn't have the right equipment on your tray

74. What is the purpose of waiting 30 seconds for the alcohol to dry before needle insertion?

    a. the evaporation process helps destroy microbes

    b. to avoid a stinging sensation

    c. to prevent hemolysis of the specimen

    d. all of the above

75. What is the *best* thing to do if the vein can be felt but not seen, even with the tourniquet on?

    a. insert the needle where you think it is and probe until you find it

    b. leave the tourniquet on while cleaning the site

    c. look for visual clues on the skin to help you remember where it is

    d. mark the spot with a felt tip pen

ANSWERS TO REVIEW QUESTIONS

1. *c.* If the needle touches the skin and then is withdrawn before piercing the tissue, the needle is considered contaminated and should be changed to avoid a possible infection.

2. *a.* As part of "informed consent," you must always inform the patient of the procedure, including the name of the test that is ordered if he or she asks. The patient also has the right to know if you are a student, but it is not in your purview to comment on the patient's prognosis or chances of recovery.

3. *b.* When identifying an inpatient, ask the patient to state his or her name. This step should be done first. If the name is correct then match the requisition with the information on the ID bracelet.

4. *d.* Ankle veins should be used as a last resort and after checking with the patient's doctor.

5. *a.* A computer-generated requisition contains an accession number given to the patient's sample during the data entry phase. Sunquest's accession numbers begin with the first letter of the day of the week in which the sample is received and then the number of the sample received that day.

6. *b.* The type of test ordered is stated as a mnemonic code with the number of tubes needed preceding the type of tube to use in collection; for example "1LAV" means obtain one lavender tube.

7. *d.* Applying pressure on the gauze while removing the needle causes the needle to tear the skin, causing pain to the patient, and slowing down the process.

8. *a.* To enhance the vein selection, you are encouraged to palpate the antecubital area, lower the arm, and use a warming device to increase the blood flow. It is not a good idea to have the patient vigorously pump his or her fist because it may cause erroneous results in a number of tests due to hemoconcentration.

9. *d.* It is not proper technique to collect specimens stopper-end first because reflux (flow of blood from the tube back into the vein) may occur. Carry-over of additives to other tubes by means of blood left in the needle as tubes are changed is another result of filling tubes from the stopper end first.

10. *b.* Grasp the patient's arm with your nondominant hand, using your thumb to pull the skin taut 1 to 2 inches below the intended site. For

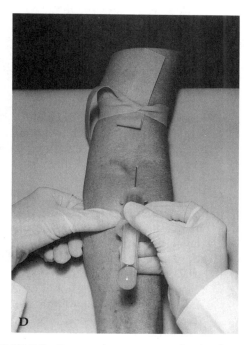

FIGURE 9-2. Entering the vein, notice the thumb drawing the skin taut (note: the tourniquet has been retied).

safety reasons, using the index finger and the thumb for anchoring the vein (two finger technique) is no longer recommended (Fig. 9-2).

11. *d.* The date and time ordered are very important to a requisition. The time is given in military time to minimize reading and transcription errors; for example, 1239 is 12:39 PM.

12. *a.* It is important that the information on the ID band match the information on the requisition exactly. The medical record number is mandatory information and should match exactly. The room number and physician may change during a patient's stay in the hospital and should not be relied on as proper ID. The test status changes with each order and cannot be used as any form of ID.

13. *b.* For normal venous punctures, the best angle is 15 to 30 degrees. When using a butterfly, the angle will probably be less than 15 degrees and if the vein is deep a sharper angle is required.

14. *c.* Do everything you can to establish a rapport with the child and his parents. Even young children can sense when you are not being honest with them. Let them know it may be slightly uncomfortable without being overly blunt. Never tell them it will not hurt.

15. *b.* Even if the ID band and the requisition matches, it is not adequate as proper identification of the patient. An ID band on the night stand could belong to a patient who previously occupied that bed. For this reason, identification should never be verified from an ID band that is *not* attached to the patient.

16. *a.* Dorsal hand vein procedure on infants does not require the use of a tourniquet.

17. *d.* Carefully slide the needle along the removal slot on the sharps container until it drops in. Do not leave sharps partially exposed or use your hands to dispose of unsheathed sharps. Shaking the sharps container can cause the needle to fly out or other sharps to come out of the container.

18. *a.* If you determine that the patient has not been fasting, the nursing staff should be informed so that a determination can be made regarding whether to proceed with the test. In the event that you are told to proceed with collection, you should write "nonfasting" on the requisition and label so that the person doing the testing knows the status of the patient.

19. *b.* The NCCLS says to clean the site using a circular motion, starting at the center of the site and moving outward in ever widening concentric circles. Use sufficient pressure to remove surface dirt and debris.

20. *d.* If the request is for a STAT or timed specimen, excuse yourself, explain why you are there, and ask permission to proceed.

21. *b.* Vigorous mixing or shaking the tube can cause hemolysis because red cells are fragile and can rupture easily.

22. *b.* Allowing pediatric patients to brace their own arms is asking for trouble. Even if it appears that they understand and will stay still, chances are they will pull away as soon as they see the needle.

23. *b.* You can tell when the needle enters the vein, you will feel a slight "give" or decrease in resistance. If the needle hisses, you know you are pulling in air and are partially or totally out of the vein. If you can feel the needle vibrate, the needle bevel is against a

vein wall and causing a flapping of the tissue against the needle opening.

24. *b.* Most patients understand that blood tests are needed in the course of their treatment. Occasionally a patient will not want to be punctured and will be rude and cranky. If this should happen, you will treat the patient in the normal way being as polite and professional as you can be.

25. *c.* To minimize the effects of stasis and hemoconcentration, the tourniquet should never be left in place longer than 1 minute. On patients with fragile veins that might collapse, or in other difficult draw situations where release of the tourniquet might cause stoppage of blood flow, the tourniquet is sometimes left on until the last tube is filled.

26. *d.* Carrying a bag or purse on the venipuncture arm, lifting heavy objects with that arm or removing the bandage prematurely can all disturb the healing process and reinitiate bleeding or cause bruising of the site.

27. *d.* When a syringe needle is inserted in a vein, a "flash" of blood will usually appear in the hub of the needle.

28. *a.* As soon as blood flows into the tube, release the tourniquet and have the patient release his or her fist. To minimize the effects of stasis and hemoconcentration, the tourniquet should never be left in place longer than 1 minute.

29. *a.* Veins can collapse if the collection tube is too large for the size of the vein, if the patient has fragile veins (common in the elderly), or if a syringe plunger is pulled too quickly while withdrawing the blood. Drawing multiple tubes on patients is common practice and as long as the tubes are proper for the size of the vein, this should not cause the vein to collapse.

30. *d.* Misidentification of a patient's specimen can be grounds for dismissal of the person responsible and could even lead to a malpractice lawsuit against that person.

31. *b.* To ensure a proper ratio of additive to blood, let the tube fill until the vacuum is exhausted and blood ceases to flow. Tubes will not fill completely. When an anticoagulant is used, the specimen will not clot. The only evacuated tube that is sensitive to tissue thromboplastin contamination is the light-blue stoppered tube.

32. *c.* Using dorsal hand vein technique to collect blood from neonates causes minimal trauma and appears to be less painful to infants than heel puncture. The toe is not an acceptable site for skin puncture on infants. Performing venipuncture on antecubital veins of newborns should be reserved for special situations, never for routine blood collection.

33. *d.* Nonadditive tubes (for example, plain red) are not mixed. In fact, mixing may cause hemolysis to occur if the sample has already begun to clot.

34. *c.* The *best* way to collect a PKU specimen from a dorsal hand vein is to let the blood drip directly onto the PKU filter paper. Blood collected in an EDTA microcollection tube or syringe may have microclots that could cause erroneous results.

35. *b.* If the tube contains an additive, mix it immediately by gently inverting it 5 to 10 times before putting it down.

36. *c.* It is not uncommon for an emergency room to receive an unconscious patient with no identification. Specimens should not be collected without some way to positively connect the specimen with the patient. In many institutions, a

phlebotomist will attach a special three-part ID band to the unidentified patient's wrist.

37. *d.* If the patient is asleep, you should wake him or her by shaking the bed, not the patient, gently. Speak softly but distinctly and avoid turning on bright lights. Never attempt to collect a blood specimen from a sleeping patient. Such an attempt may startle the patient and cause injury to the patient or you.

38. *b.* The arm should be supported firmly and extended downward in a straight line from the shoulder to the wrist. The arm should not be bent at the elbow.

39. *d.* To avoid continued bleeding and bruising, do not allow the patient to fold his or her arm after venipuncture. A gauze pad in a folded arm may not apply direct pressure to the site and when the arm is opened, the platelet plug can be dislodged.

40. *a.* If the needle bevel is not completely under the skin and the tube is fully advanced onto the needle, the tube will lose its vacuum as evidenced by a hissing sound. A tube that has lost its vacuum will no longer fill with blood and must be replaced with a new one.

41. *c.* A big factor in successful blood collection from pediatric patients is proper immobilization. Preventing excessive movement makes the process quicker and safer for the patient as well as the blood drawer.

42. *d.* Never say, "Are you Mr. Jones?" A person who is very ill, hard of hearing, or on heavy medication may say "yes" to anything.

43. *d.* When the tube is advanced past the guideline on the holder, the stopper is penetrated causing the tube to lose the vacuum which means it will not fill and must be replace by a new tube.

44. *d.* Specimen tube labels should contain all of the following information as a minimum: first and last name, hospital number or date of birth, and phlebotomist's initials. The room number and bed may be found on the label if the label has been generated by a computer, but is not mandatory.

45. *a.* Outpatients do not normally have ID bands and verifying identification by a name tag from the patient's place of employment is not adequate. You should ask an outpatient his or her name and date of birth.

46. *d.* The patient's ID number is included on the specimen label to avoid confusing samples. It is not unusual to have patients with the same or similar names in the hospital at the same time, but two patients will not have the same hospital or medical record number.

47. *c.* The biggest advantage of using a butterfly is the ability to collect blood specimens from small and difficult veins.

48. *a.* Sclerosed veins feel hard and cord-like, lacking resiliency. They are difficult to penetrate and roll easily.

49. *d.* Visually inspecting the needle tip before insertion not only ensures that you are entering bevel up, but also prevents damage and unnecessary pain during the procedure should the point or beveled edges have imperfections. Outdated needles must be removed from the stock during regular inventory of the stock.

50. *d.* The test collection process begins when the physician orders or "requests" a test to be performed on a patient. All laboratory testing must be requested by a physician and results reported to a physician.

51. *b.* During a multiple tube draw it is possible for the additive of a tube to

be carried over to the tube that follows. It has been demonstrated that carryover of sodium or potassium EDTA can grossly contaminate subsequently drawn tubes, especially affecting those for electrolyte determination. For this reason, NCCLS recommends that EDTA (lavender stopper) tubes be collected after heparin (green stopper) tubes. If you should forget and fill the EDTA before the green, you should draw a discard tube to remove EDTA contamination before drawing the green stopper.

52. *c.* When an evacuated tube has been filled as full as possible, the pressure in the tube and needle will be equalized and blood remaining in the needle will drip out as it is being put in a sharps container. The last tube should be removed from the holder before withdrawing the needle to reduce the risk of blood contamination on all adjacent surfaces.

53. *c.* Small children seldom hold still for blood collection. The flexibility of the butterfly tubing enables successful blood collection despite some movement by the child.

54. *a.* Inpatient blood specimens should be labeled at the bedside immediately following collection. If tubes are labeled before collection and one of the tubes is not used at that time, another patient's blood could end up in that labeled tube. If tubes are labeled away from the bedside, the specimen can be misidentified.

55. *a.* You should apply the tourniquet three to four inches above the intended venipuncture site. A position farther away would minimize the effect of the tourniquet (Fig. 9-3). A tourniquet tied too close

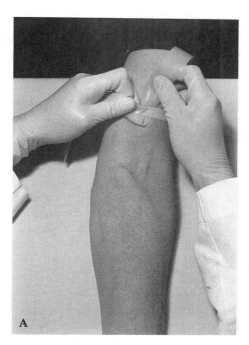

FIGURE 9-3. Applying the tourniquet.

to the site may cause the vein to collapse during blood collection. A tourniquet is never applied below the collection site.

56. *d.* A tourniquet that is tied too tightly may prevent arterial blood flow into the area resulting in failure to get the blood. When a tourniquet is too tight, it will pinch and hurt the patient and cause the arm to turn red or purple resulting in hemoconcentration and changing the results of the sample.

57. *a.* The most important step in specimen collection is patient identification. Applying the tourniquet, selecting the correct specimen tube, and handling the specimen properly are all very important in quality assurance. But, if a specimen is obtained from the wrong patient, it can have serious, even fatal consequences.

58. *c.* If a butterfly needle is barely in the vein it may spin around and pull out when the phlebotomist lets go of it. In addition, the needle bevel may be only partly in the vein causing the vein to "blow" or a hematoma to quickly form. Slightly threading the needle along the central area (lumen) of the vein will help anchor the needle in the vein.

59. *a.* If the door to the room is closed, you should knock lightly and proceed with caution. Even if the door is open, it is a good idea to knock lightly to make occupants aware that you are about to enter.

60. *d.* Lack of or inadequate mixing immediately after filling anticoagulant tubes can lead to microclot formation. Nonadditive tubes do not require mixing.

61. *a.* Older children appreciate honesty and will be more cooperative if you explain what you are going to do and stress the importance of holding still.

62. *a.* You should remain calm and treat the patient as you would a fearful adult. Explain the procedure in simple terms and ask for the child's cooperation.

63. *c.* When it has been determined that a patient truly refuses to cooperate, you should write on the requisition that the patient has refused to have blood drawn. You should also notify the patient's nurse and the phlebotomy supervisor that the specimen was not obtained because of patient refusal.

64. *d.* After the last tube has been filled and removed from the holder, a clean gauze square is folded in fourths and placed directly over the needle without pressing down. As the needle is removed from the arm, immediate pressure is applied to the site for 3 to 5 minutes. The folded gauze pad allows for more pressure to be applied directly to the site preventing leakage of blood and hematoma formation.

65. *b.* When performing a routine blood draw, the hands must be washed before glove application at the beginning of the procedure and at the end, before proceeding to the next patient.

66. *c.* When transferring blood from a syringe to an evacuated tube, place the tube in a rack before penetrating the tube stopper with the needle. Holding the tube in your hand is dangerous because the needle may slip and stick your hand. Let the vacuum of the tube draw the blood into it. Pushing on the plunger and forcing blood into the tube it can hemolyze the specimen and can also allow blood to spurt out around the needle and contaminate you.

67. *b.* Proper blood collection technique requires that the needle be centered in the vein. Blood cannot be successfully collected when the needle has penetrated all the way through the vein or the tube has lost its vacuum. Blood will not flow into the tube properly when the needle is only partially inserted in the vein.

68. *d.* Usually such inquiries are handled by stating that the doctor has ordered the tests as part of the patient's care and that the doctor will be happy to explain the tests to him or her if asked.

69. *c.* Gauze pads are preferred to cotton balls when applying pressure to the puncture site because the cotton fibers can get entwined in the clot formation and dislodge the platelet plug when removed.

70. *b.* Identification should never be based on the room number and patient's name on the appropriate door. When no ID band can be found, it is necessary to ask the patient's nurse to make positive identification and attach an ID band before the specimen can be drawn. In case of an emergency where the patient has no ID band, the phlebotomist may ask the patient's nurse to initial the requisition before preceeding.

71. *d.* A used, unsheathed needle can be thought of as a weapon and should not be carried across the room or held in the air until it is possible to dispose of it properly in a sharps container. Resheathing the needle using a one-handed method is acceptable in this circumstance to avoid an accidental puncture by a dirty needle.

72. *a.* When the blood-drawing needle is only partially inserted in the vein, the tube will fill very slowly and blood will leak into the tissue around the vein causing a hematoma.

73. *d.* Patient refusal or unavailability, or the fact that you tried but were unsuccessful are all valid reasons for failure to obtain specimen. Not having the right equipment to collect a specimen makes a phlebotomist appear disorganized and unprofessional and is *not* an acceptable reason for failure to collect a specimen. You should check to see that you have the proper equipment for the test before leaving to collect the specimen.

74. *d.* The "30-second waiting time" after cleansing with alcohol serves many purposes. Besides helping to destroy microbes on the skin, it prevents hemolysis of the specimen and the stinging sensation when penetrating the site through alcohol.

75. *c.* If the vein can be felt, but not seen, try to mentally visualize the location. It often helps to note the position of the vein in reference to a mole, hair, or skin crease.

Skin Puncture

10

REVIEW QUESTIONS

1. A blood smear made from an EDTA specimen should be made:
   a. within 1 hour of collection
   b. within 4 hours of collection
   c. within 12 hours after collection
   d. anytime after collection

2. The most common site for skin puncture on children 2 years of age or older is the:
   a. bottom of the ear lobe
   b. fleshy side of the thumb
   c. palmar fleshy portion of the finger
   d. plantar medial portion of the heel

3. Which of the following is *not* proper finger puncture procedure?
   a. avoid squeezing or vigorous massaging
   b. puncture parallel to the "whorls" of the fingerprint
   c. puncture the middle or ring finger
   d. wipe away the first drop of blood

4. Why is it inappropriate to apply a bandage to skin puncture sites of infants less than 2 years of age?
   a. adhesive bandages irritate their tender skin
   b. the bandage may come off and be a choking hazard for the infant
   c. the bandage may tear the skin when removed
   d. all of the above

5. Which of the following devices should *never* be used for skin puncture?
   a. autolet
   b. metal lancet
   c. surgical blade
   d. Tenderlett®

6. Which of the following is a proper site for a fingerstick on an adult?
   a. distal phalanx of the middle or ring finger
   b. distal phalanx of the thumb
   c. medial phalanx of the right index finger

   d. proximal phalanx of the middle or ring finger

7. Allow alcohol to dry before performing skin puncture to avoid:
   a. hematoma
   b. hemoconcentration
   c. hemolysis
   d. hemostasis

8. A microcollection reservoir that contains a fluid for direct dilution of the specimen is a:
   a. capillary tube
   b. microtainer
   c. Natelson tube
   d. Unopette®

9. Why are capillary blood gases less desirable than arterial blood gases (ABGs)?
   a. skin puncture blood contains tissue fluid
   b. skin puncture blood is only partly arterial in composition
   c. the blood is exposed to air during collection
   d. all of the above

10. What is the National Committee for Clinical Laboratory Standards (NCCLS) recommended maximum depth of puncture to be used during heel puncture?
    a. 1.0 mm
    b. 1.4 mm
    c. 2.4 mm
    d. 2.8 mm

11. Why are blood smears and EDTA specimens obtained before other specimens when collected by skin puncture?
    a. collection order does not matter
    b. to minimize effects of platelet clumping
    c. to minimize tissue fluid contamination
    d. to reduce effects of hemolysis

12. Why should a laboratory report form indicate the fact that a specimen has been collected by skin puncture?
    a. because test results may vary depending on the method of collection
    b. for liability insurance and billing purposes
    c. so that subsequent specimens will be collected by skin puncture also
    d. so that the patient's nurse can check the site for signs of infection

13. Which test is most affected by alcohol residue?
    a. blood urea nitrogen
    b. capillary blood gases
    c. glucose
    d. potassium

14. Which statement is *not* true? Capillary blood gases:
    a. are more accurate than ABGs
    b. are performed on infants because arterial puncture is too dangerous
    c. contain both venous and arterial system blood
    d. use an open collection system

15. The following tests are ordered on the same patient. If skin puncture is used, which specimen should be collected first?
    a. bilirubin
    c. CBC
    d. glucose
    e. lytes

16. Which of the following is the safest area for infant heel puncture? The:
    a. area of the arch
    b. central area
    c. lateral plantar surface
    d. posterior curvature

17. Iron filings used when collecting capillary blood gases:
    a. aid in mixing the anticoagulant
    b. keep the blood from sticking to the sides of the tube
    c. prevent air bubble formation
    d. react with oxygen to stabilize the specimen

18. A skin puncture should be done rather than a venipuncture in all of the following situations except:
    a. a child less than 2 years of age
    b. a patient with difficult veins
    c. when a light-blue stoppered tube is needed
    d. when a small volume of blood is adequate

19. Which of the following is a newborn screening test?
    a. activated coagulation time (ACT)
    b. bilirubin
    c. phenylketonuria (PKU)
    d. white blood cell count

20. The purpose of wiping away the first drop of blood during skin puncture is to:
    a. avoid bacterial contamination
    b. eliminate tissue fluid contamination
    c. minimize effects of hemolysis
    d. minimize effects of platelet aggregation

21. Skin puncture blood most closely resembles:
    a. arterial blood
    b. intracellular fluid
    c. tissue fluid
    d. venous blood

22. What does the term "calcaneus" mean?
    a. bone infection
    b. calcium containing
    c. heel bone
    d. osteomyelitis

23. Skin puncture blood reference values (normals) are higher for:
    a. calcium
    b. glucose
    c. phosphorous
    d. total protein

24. To lengthen a smear that is too short, the phlebotomist should try again and:
    a. exert more pressure with the spreader slide
    b. decrease the angle of the spreader slide
    c. increase the angle of the spreader slide
    d. use a smaller drop of blood

25. Which of the following is a test performed on newborns to detect inability to metabolize an amino acid?
    a. bilirubin
    b. CBC
    c. PKU
    d. T_4

26. Which microcollection container would be used to collect a CBC?
    a. gray
    b. green
    c. lavender
    d. red

27. Which of the following tests requires warming of the heel before specimen collection for accurate results?
    a. bilirubin
    b. blood gases
    c. electrolytes
    d. PKU

28. What is PKU?
    a. a contagious condition caused by lack of phenylalanine
    b. a hereditary inability to metabolize phenylalanine
    c. an acquired condition caused by lack of phenylalanine
    d. an inherited condition caused by lack of thyroid hormone

29. Which of the following can be a complication resulting from deep skin punctures of an infant's heel?
    a. anemia
    b. hepatitis
    c. osteochondritis
    d. phenylketonuria

30. Contamination of a PKU test can result from:
    a. failure to discard first drop
    b. presence of alcohol residue
    c. touching blood spot circles before or after collection
    d. all of the above

31. It is necessary to control depth of lancet insertion during skin puncture in order to avoid:
    a. bacterial contamination
    b. bone injury
    c. excessive bleeding
    d. puncturing an artery

32. An acceptable smear:
    a. covers the entire surface of the slide
    b. forms a bullet shape
    c. has a feathered uniform edge
    d. is short and thick

33. Which of the following most accurately describes skin puncture blood? Skin puncture blood is:
    a. a mixture of venous, arterial, and capillary blood
    b. is mostly tissue fluid mixed with arterial blood
    c. mostly venous blood and tissue fluid
    d. nearly identical to venous blood

34. Which of the following microcollection tubes is sometimes used as a hematology screening test?
    a. Caraway
    b. large-bore capillary
    c. microhematocrit
    d. Natelson

35. Which of the following equipment *may* be required to collect capillary blood gases?
    a. magnet
    b. metal flea
    c. warming device
    d. all of the above

36. Which of the following would be eliminated as a skin puncture site?
    a. an edematous extremity
    b. a site below an intravenous catheter
    c. the lateral plantar surface of a baby's heel
    d. the middle or ring finger of a warm adult hand

37. The capillary bed from which skin puncture blood is obtained is located in the:
    a. dermis and subcutaneous junction
    b. junction of the dermis and epidermis
    c. lower epidermis
    d. upper dermis only

38. Which of the following makes up the largest portion of skin puncture blood?
    a. arterial blood
    b. intracellular fluid
    c. tissue fluid
    d. venous blood

39. What is the purpose of warming the site before skin puncture?
    a. it increases blood flow up to 7 times
    b. it makes the veins more visible
    c. the warmth comforts the patient
    d. to prevent hemolysis of the sample

40. Which of the following equipment is *not* used to collect skin puncture specimens?
    a. capillary tubes
    b. evacuated tubes
    c. lancets
    d. microsampler

ANSWERS TO REVIEW QUESTIONS

1. *a.* A blood smear when made from an EDTA-anticoagulated blood should be made within one hour of collection to eliminate cell distortion caused by the anticoagulant.

2. *c.* The recommended site for skin puncture on older children is the palmar surface of the end segment, fleshy portion of the finger.

3. *b.* To perform a proper finger puncture one should puncture the middle or ring finger perpendicularly to the "whorls" of the fingerprint (Fig. 10-1).

4. *d.* Bandages should not be applied to skin puncture sites of infants under two years of age because adhesive bandages may irritate their tender skin or tear the skin when removed, in addition the bandage could come off and be a choking hazard.

5. *c.* A metal lancet, the Autolet, and the Tenderlett are all devices that have been designed to puncture a

prescribed, safe depth (Fig. 10-2). The surgical blade was not designed for skin puncture and, if used, can penetrate the tissue all the way to the bone.

6. *a.* The recommended site for skin puncture on an adult is the palmar surface of the distal phalanx (end segment of the finger) of the middle or ring finger of the non-dominant hand.

7. *c.* If the alcohol is not allowed to dry before performing skin puncture the specimen may be hemolyzed. Wiping the first drop of blood collected eliminates alcohol residue that could cause hemolysis and tissue fluid contamination from the first drop as well.

8. *d.* Unopettes® (Fig. 10-3) are microcollection reservoirs that contain fluid for direct dilution of specimens for hematology. Capillary and Natelson tubes which

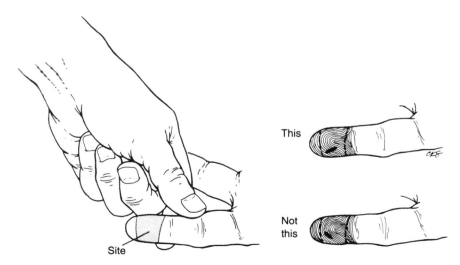

FIGURE 10-1. Recommended site and direction of finger puncture.

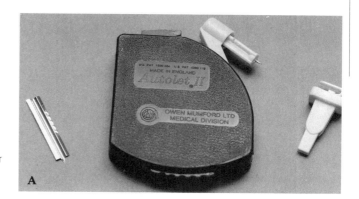

FIGURE 10-2. Metal lancet; Autolet (Ulster Scientific Inc., New Paltz, NY); Safety Flow Lancet (Becton Dickinson, Franklin Lakes, NJ).

fill by capillary action are used for hematocrits and capillary blood gases, respectively. Microtainers are small tubes that are color-coded like evacuated tubes and are used for collection of hematology and chemistry tests.

9. *d.* Skin puncture blood is less desirable for blood gases because of its partial arterial composition and contamination with tissue fluid, but also because it is temporarily exposed to air during collection. All of these could possibly alter blood gas results.

10. *c.* According to NCCLS, the recommended maximum depth of puncture to be used during heel puncture is 2.4 mm. Studies have shown that the calcaneus of premature infants may be as little as 2.4 mm below the skin surface on the bottom of the heel and half that distance at the back of the heel.

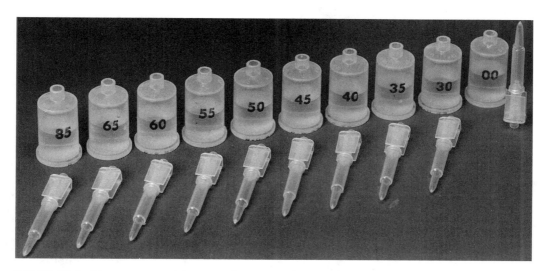

FIGURE 10-3. Unopette system (Courtesy of Becton Dickinson and Co., Franklin Lakes, NJ).

11. *b.* Immediately after puncturing the skin, platelets begin to aggregate or clump to close the puncture site. If hematology tests, such as, blood smears, need to be collected they must be obtained first to avoid erroneous results due to increased platelet counts.

12. *a.* Skin puncture blood differs in composition from regular venous blood; therefore, the fact that a specimen has been collected by skin puncture should be indicated on the laboratory report form.

13. *d.* Alcohol residue interferes with glucose testing.

14. *a.* Capillary blood gases are less accurate than arterial blood gases because they contain both venous and arterial system blood and they are exposed to air during collection. However, they are performed on infants because arterial puncture is too dangerous.

15. *c.* Hematology tests, such as a CBC, need to be collected first to avoid erroneous results due to increased platelet counts. Bilirubin, glucose and lytes are usually collected in a red microtainer, allowed to clot and, therefore, are not affected by platelet aggregation.

16. *c.* As established by NCCLS guidelines, heel punctures should only be performed on the plantar surface of the heel, lateral to an imaginary line extending from between the fourth and fifth toes to the heel (Fig. 10-4).

17. *a.* Iron filings, often referred to as "fleas," are inserted into the tube after collection of a capillary blood gas specimen to aid in mixing the anticoagulant.

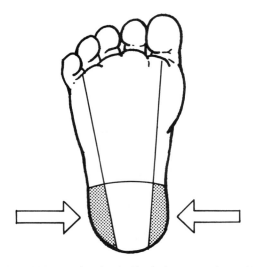

FIGURE 10-4. Infant heel. Shaded areas indicated by arrows represent recommended areas for infant heel puncture.

18. *c.* Some tests cannot be performed on skin puncture specimens. One of these is coagulation studies which must be collected in a light blue stopper tube.

19. *c.* Newborn screening is performed to test for the presence of genetic or inherited disease, the most common of which is PKU or phenylketonuria.

20. *b.* Always wipe away the first drop of blood (Fig. 10-5) during skin puncture because the first drop is usually contaminated with tissue fluids which can effect test results.

21. *a.* Skin puncture blood contains arterial and venous blood along with small amounts of intracellular and tissue fluid. It is more arterial in composition due to the pressure with which arterial blood enters the capillaries and therefore more closely resembles arterial blood.

22. *c.* The calcaneus is the heel bone and is located at the back and bottom on the foot.

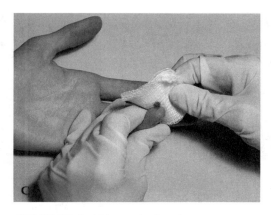

FIGURE 10-5. Wiping the first drop.

23. *b.* Normal or reference values for certain tests will be different for skin puncture blood; the most notable differences are for glucose, which is higher in skin puncture blood.

24. *b.* Smears that are too short or too long are not acceptable. The length of the smear can be controlled by the size of the drop and the angle of the spreader slide. If a phlebotomist wishes to lengthen a smear, he/she should decrease the angle of the spreader slide.

25. *c.* The PKU test is performed on newborns to detect inability to metabolize the amino acid phenylalanine.

26. *c.* The lavender microcollection container used for CBCs is the same color-code as the evacuated tubes used for hematology tests.

27. *b.* Collection of blood gases on infants requires warming of the heel prior to specimen collection because warming increases blood flow to the site or arterializes the specimen. Warming the site makes collection of bilirubin, electrolytes and PKU specimens easier, but is not required for accuracy of results.

28. *b.* PKU is a hereditary disease caused by the inability of the body to metabolize phenylalanine due to a defective enzyme. Mental retardation results if not treated early.

29. *c.* Puncture of the bone can cause osteochondritis or inflammation of the bone and cartilage.

30. *d.* Since PKUs are collected by placing one large drop of blood on filter paper, they can easily be contaminated if the first drop of blood is not wiped away, if there is presence of alcohol residue on the skin, or if the circles have been touched preventing them from absorbing properly.

31. *b.* Bone injury is a concern when performing skin puncture. For this reason, guidelines have been developed by NCCLS recommending where skin punctures should be performed.

32. *c.* An acceptable blood smear should cover about one-half the surface of the slide and have the appearance of a feather in that there will be a smooth gradient from thick to thin when held up to the light (Fig. 10-6).

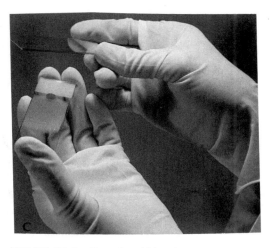

FIGURE 10-6. Completed blood smear.

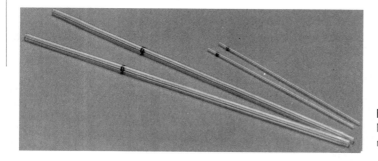

FIGURE 10-7. Microcollection tubes: Natelson tubes on the left and microhematocrit tubes on the right.

33. *a.* Blood obtained through skin puncture is a mixture of arterial blood, venous blood and capillary blood, along with interstitial and intracellular fluids from the surrounding tissues.

34. *c.* A microhematocrit tube is sometimes used for a hematology screening test called a hematocrit (Fig. 10-7).

35. *d.* Equipment required to collect capillary blood gases includes a magnet and metal flea for mixing the blood after collection and a warming device used to arterialize the specimen (Fig. 10-8).

36. *a.* A skin puncture, as well as a venipuncture, may be performed on a site below an IV. A skin puncture performed on an edematous extremity will result in erroneous results due to increase tissue fluid in the sample.

37. *a.* The dermis contains blood and lymph vessels. These structures also extend into the subcutaneous layer; therefore, it is said that the capillary bed is located at the junction of the dermis and epidermis.

38. *a.* Skin puncture blood contains both venous and arterial blood along with

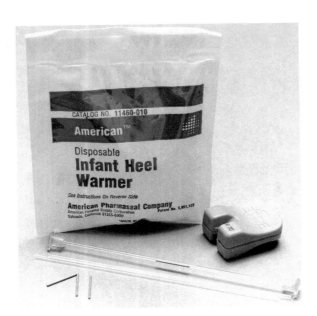

FIGURE 10-8. Capillary blood gas equipment.

a small amount of fluid from the cells and tissues. However, it contains a higher proportion of arterial blood than venous blood because of the pressure with which the arterial blood enters the capillaries.

39. *a.* Blood flow can be increased up to seven times by warming the site

prior to skin puncture. This warming primarily increases arterial flow and is said to "arterialize" the specimen.

40. *b.* Skin puncture equipment includes capillary tubes, microtainers, and lancets. Evacuated tubes are used in venipuncture collections.

Special Procedures and Point-of-Care Testing

11

A. **Special Venipuncture Procedures**
   1. Blood Alcohol (Ethanol) Specimens
   2. Forensic Specimens
   3. Blood Bank Specimens for Type and Crossmatch
   4. Blood Donor Collection
      a. Donor Eligibility
      b. Procedure
   5. Autologous Blood Donations
   6. Blood Cultures
   7. Postprandial Glucose Testing
   8. Glucose Tolerance Test
   9. Other Tolerance Tests
      a. Lactose Tolerance Test
      b. Epinephrine Tolerance Test
      c. Glucagon Tolerance Test
   10. Trace Metals
   11. Therapeutic Drug Monitoring
   12. Therapeutic Phlebotomy
B. **Point-of-Care Testing**
   1. Activated Coagulation Time
   2. Bleeding Time
   3. Blood Gases
   4. Chemistry Panel
   5. Cholesterol/High-Density (HDL)/ Low-Density Lipoprotein (LDL)
   6. Glucose
   7. Hemoglobin/Hematocrit
   8. Ionized Calcium
   9. Occult Blood
   10. Skin Tests
      a. Types
         (1) Tuberculin (TB) Test
         (2) Shick Test
         (3) Dick Test
         (4) Histoplasmosis (Histo) Test
         (5) Coccidioidomycosis (Cocci) Test
      b. Procedure
      c. Interpretation
   11. Urinalysis
      a. Dipstick
      b. Pregnancy

REVIEW QUESTIONS

1. Sources of error for point-of-care testing for blood-glucose monitoring are all of the following *except*:
   a. inadequate sample size
   b. patient's hematocrit between 25% and 60%
   c. dehydrated patient
   d. elevated bilirubin count

2. Which of the following tests must be collected using special skin decontamination procedures?

a. blood cultures
b. blood urea nitrogen
c. complete blood count
d. type and crossmatch

3. A bleeding time (BT) test assesses the functioning of which cellular element?
   a. erythrocytes
   b. leukocytes
   c. neutrophils
   d. thrombocytes

4. What type additive is *best* for collecting an ethanol test?
   a. EDTA
   b. nonadditive red stopper
   c. sodium citrate
   d. sodium fluoride

5. When reading a patient's TB test, there is an area of induration and erythema that measures 7 mm in diameter. The result of the test is:
   a. doubtful
   b. negative
   c. positive
   d. unreadable

6. A "peak" TDM level has been ordered for 0900. You draw the specimen *10* minutes late because of unavoidable circumstances. What additional action does this necessitate?
   a. establish the last dosage time
   b. notify the patient's nurse
   c. record time change when verifying collection
   d. all of the above

7. Of the following analytes, which cannot be measured through point-of-care testing on a hand-held instrument, such as I-Stat?
   a. bicarbonate
   b. chloride
   c. hematocrit
   d. phosphorus

8. Which blood culture container should be inoculated first when the specimen has been collected by syringe?

a. aerobic
b. anaerobic
c. either
d. neither

9. What does induration mean?
   a. hardness
   b. necrotic
   c. redness
   d. warm

10. Which are eligibility requirements for donating blood?
    a. age 17 to 66 years, 110 lb or more, good health
    b. age 18 to 75 years, good health, 110 lb
    c. at least 100 lb, 21 to 65 years old, good health
    d. minimum of age 21 years, no risky behavior, good health

11. What special equipment is needed to draw an activated coagulation time (ACT)?
    a. blood pressure cuff, heat block
    b. blood pressure cuff, stopwatch or timer
    c. stopwatch or timer, incubator or heat block
    d. stopwatch or timer, povidone iodine solution

12. Failure to draw a discard tube before ACT collection may:
    a. decrease clotting time because of tissue thromboplastin contamination
    b. decrease clotting time because of platelet plug formation
    c. increase clotting time because of alcohol residue contamination
    d. none of the above

13. How much antigen is injected when performing a purified protein derivative (PPD) test?
    a. 0.01 mL
    b. 0.1 mL
    c. 1.0 mL
    d. 10 mL

14. Glucose levels 30 minutes after epinephrine stimulation increase more than 30 mg/dL over fasting levels. This indicates that the patient has:
    a. adequate liver glycogen stores
    b. diabetes mellitus
    c. inadequate liver glycogen stores
    d. von Gierke's disease

15. At what intervals is the blood blotted during a bleeding time test?
    a. 10 seconds
    b. 20 seconds
    c. 30 seconds
    d. 60 seconds

16. Which of the following tests is collected from patients with fever of unknown origin (FUO) to rule out septicemia?
    a. blood culture
    b. nasopharyngeal cultures
    c. urine culture and sensitivity (C & S)
    d. wound culture

17. When performing a bleeding time test, the sphygmomanometer should be inflated to:
    a. 40 mm Hg
    b. 60 mm Hg
    c. 100 mm Hg
    d. a sphygmomanometer is not needed

18. Which of the following can be used to clean a site before blood alcohol collection?
    a. isopropanol
    b. methanol
    c. tincture of iodine
    d. Zephiran chloride

19. Which of the following can affect glucose levels?
    a. chewing sugarless gum
    b. drinking tea without sugar
    c. smoking low tar cigarettes
    d. all of the above

20. Glycosuria is frequently detected by which of the following methods?
    a. AccuMeter
    b. I-Stat
    c. One-Touch
    d. urine dipstick

21. This test can determine if a person has produced antibodies to a particular antigen.
    a. gastric analysis
    b. glucose tolerance test (GTT)
    c. skin test
    d. Hollander test

22. Which of the following tests detects occult blood in feces?
    a. gastric analysis
    b. guaiac
    c. PPD
    d. Schick

23. When does the specimen timing of a GTT begin?
    a. a GTT is not timed
    b. after the fasting specimen is drawn
    c. after the patient has finished the glucose beverage
    d. before the fasting specimen is drawn

24. Which of the following is a skin test for tuberculosis exposure?
    a. cocci
    b. histo
    c. PPD
    d. Shick

25. Which of the following tests may require special "chain of custody" documentation when collected?
    a. blood culture
    b. crossmatch
    c. drug screen
    d. TDM

26. What constitutes a positive skin test?
    a. any amount of erythema
    b. induration and erythema less than 5 mm
    c. erythema and induration of 5 to 9 mm
    d. erythema and induration 10 mm or greater

27. Name a condition in which a unit of blood is withdrawn from a patient as a treatment?
    a. autologous donation
    b. ABO Rh incompatibility

c. leukemia
d. polycythemia

28. What does the term "erythema" mean?
    a. hardness
    b. irritation
    c. redness
    d. swelling

29. In which instrument is the blood placed in a microcuvette rather than on a test strip for glucose testing?
    a. AccuChek®
    b. Glucometer®
    c. HemoCue®
    d. One-Touch II®

30. Which type of test requires special identification and labeling procedures?
    a. BUN
    b. CBC
    c. PT
    d. T & C

31. Which of the following will *not* affect a bleeding time?
    a. an abnormally low platelet count
    b. inflating the sphygmomanometer to 40 mm Hg
    c. ingestion of aspirin-containing drugs
    d. touching the incision with the blotting paper

32. Which type tube is needed to collect blood for T & C?
    a. gray plain
    b. plain red
    c. royal blue
    d. serum separator tube (SST)

33. Which of the following equipment is *not* needed for a bleeding time test?
    a. butterfly bandage
    b. standardized incision device
    c. stopwatch
    d. tourniquet

34. An autologous blood transfusion is a transfusion of blood:
    a. directly from donor to patient
    b. donated by the patient for his or her own use

c. donated from a relative
d. from an anonymous donor

35. The most critical aspect of blood culture collection is?
    a. needle gauge
    b. volume of blood collected
    c. specimen handling
    d. skin antisepsis

36. Which point-of-care test requires a visual evaluation to determine the end point?
    a. AccuMeter®
    b. Hemacue®
    c. IRMA®
    d. I-Stat®

37. Which of the following tests would not be subject to TDM?
    a. digoxin
    b. gentamicin
    c. phenylalanine
    d. theophylline

38. In urine pregnancy testing, the hormone analyzed is:
    a. ACTH
    b. HCT
    c. HCG
    d. TSH

39. Anaerobic means:
    a. air loving
    b. no exercise
    c. room air
    d. without air

40. What type of specimen is needed for a guaiac test?
    a. amniotic fluid
    b. blood
    c. feces
    d. urine

41. The most commonly recommended antiseptic for blood culture collection is:
    a. 0.5% sodium hypochlorite
    b. 70% isopropanol
    c. povidone iodine
    d. chlorhexidene gluconate

42. Monitoring blood coagulation through point-of-care testing is performed for all of the following *except*:

a. heparin therapy
b. lithium therapy
c. transfusion therapy
d. warfarin therapy

43. Which of the following additives is used for an ACT test?
   a. EDTA
   b. heparin
   c. siliceous earth or celite
   d. sodium citrate

44. A 2-hour PP is often used as a screening test for what condition?
   a. carbohydrate metabolism problems
   b. coagulation problems
   c. fever of unknown origin
   d. malabsorption problems

45. Which of the following is a test of platelet plug formation in the capillaries?
   a. ACT
   b. BT
   c. CBC
   d. PT

46. The purpose of a lactose tolerance test is to check for:
   a. adequacy of insulin levels
   b. malabsorption in the intestines
   c. presence of the enzyme needed to metabolize milk sugar
   d. production of stomach acid

47. A patient undergoing a glucose tolerance test vomits within 30 minutes of drinking the glucose beverage. What action should the phlebotomist take?
   a. continue the test and note on the requisition that the patient vomited the solution and at what time
   b. discontinue the test and write on the requisition that the patient vomited the glucose beverage
   c. give the patient another dose of glucose beverage

d. immediately notify the patient's physician or nurse to determine if the test should be continued or rescheduled

48. Which of the following is a common "bedside test"?
   a. bilirubin
   b. glucose
   c. rapid plasma reagin
   d. serum glutamic-oxaloacetic transaminase

49. The purpose of TDM is to:
   a. determine a beneficial dose of drug for a patient
   b. maintain "peak" levels of a drug in a patient's system
   c. maintain "trough" levels of drug in a patient
   d. screen for illegal drug use

50. The phlebotomist arrives to collect a 2-hour postprandial glucose test and discovers that 2 hours have not elapsed since the patient's meal. What should the phlebotomist do?
   a. ask the patient's nurse to verify the correct time to draw the specimen
   b. come back later at the time the patient says is correct
   c. draw the specimen and write the time drawn on the specimen label
   d. fill out an incident report form and return to the laboratory

51. Why would blood cultures be collected with antimicrobial adsorbing resin?
   a. the patient has fever spikes
   b. the patient is on a broad-spectrum antibiotic
   c. to eliminate normal flora contamination
   d. remove bacterial contamination

ANSWERS TO REVIEW QUESTIONS

1. *b.* For accurate results a patient's hematocrit must be between 25% and 60%. Most instruments will default if the test area is not completely covered with sample. A dehydrated patient will have erroneous results caused by hemoconcentration. An elevated bilirubin will interfere with the testing process.

2. *a.* Blood cultures are performed to determine the presence of organisms in the blood. Special skin decontamination procedures using povidone iodine are followed to assure collection of a sterile specimen.

3. *d.* Thrombocytes or platelets are assessed using the BT test. After the incision to the arm is made, the blood flow is blotted every 30 seconds until the blood no longer stains the filter paper. The time recorded represents the activity of the platelets.

4. *d.* The antiglycolytic agent, sodium fluoride, is the best additive for collecting an ethanol test because it slows the metabolism of the specimen and preserves the analyte to be tested.

5. *a.* Results of a TB test are reported as doubtful if the area of redness or induration is between 5 mm and 9 mm in diameter. The test is negative if there is no reaction or the area of redness or induration is less than 5 mm in diameter. A TB test is positive if the area of induration and erythema is 10 mm or greater.

6. *d.* After you have drawn the specimen 10 minutes late, it is imperative that you record the time change when verifying collection. The pharmacist calculates the dosage based on the blood level values drawn at a specified time. If a specimen is drawn late, the pharmacist needs to know the exact time in order to calculate correct peak and trough levels.

7. *d.* At this time there is no point-of-care instrument that measures phosphorous. Bicarbonate, chloride, and hematocrit testing can all be performed on an I-Stat.

8. *b.* When blood cultures are collected by syringe, the anaerobic bottle is inoculated first.

9. *b.* Induration means hardness and is used in the interpretation of intradermal skin test reactions. An antibody response to a skin test results in an area of redness often accompanied by a hardness of tissue or lump.

10. *a.* To donate blood, a person must be within the ages of 17 and 66 years, weigh at least 110 pounds, and be in good health.

11. *c.* Special equipment needed to draw an ACT, besides the special gray top tube, is a stopwatch or timer and incubator or heat block. As soon as the tube is drawn, it is placed in a heat block for 60 seconds and inspected every 5 seconds thereafter until there is visible clot formation. Automated machines, such as the Hemachron machine (Fig. 11-1) that incorporate a timer, incubator, mixer and clot detector in one portable unit can also be used to perform ACTs.

12. *a.* Failure to draw a discard tube before ACT collection may decrease the clotting time because of the

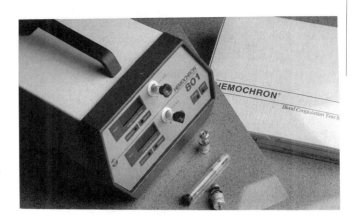

FIGURE 11-1. The Hemachron® machine for ACT determinations. (Courtesy of International Technidyne, Edison, NJ.)

introduction of tissue thromboplastin contamination into the specimen. Thromboplastin, a clot activator, will interfere with correct results and effect the heparin therapy prescribed by the physician.

13. *b.* 0.1 mL of PPD antigen is injected subcutaneously under the skin to test for antibodies to TB.

14. *a.* In a patient with normal glycogen stores, blood glucose levels at 30 minutes will increase at least 30 mg/dL above fasting levels. Little or no increase in blood sugar levels indicates inadequate liver glycogen stores or an interference in the conversion of available glycogen store, such as caused by von Gierke's disease. Epinephrine stimulation

results do not aid in the diagnosis of diabetes.

15. *c.* After the incision in the arm is made, the blood flow is blotted every 30 seconds by bringing the filter paper close to the incision and "wicking" the blood onto the filter paper without touching the wound. Touching the wound will disturb the platelet plug.

16. *a.* Blood cultures are ordered by the physician when there is "fever of unknown origin" or reason to suspect septicemia which is pathogenic bacteria in the blood (Fig. 11-2).

17. *a.* A blood pressure cuff is inflated to 40 mm Hg before the incision is

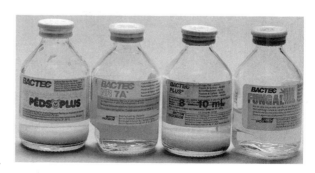

FIGURE 11-2. Blood culture bottles.

made and the pressure is maintained throughout the entire procedure for standardization purposes.

18. *d.* A non–alcohol-containing antiseptic such as Zephiran chloride (a trade name for benzalkonium chloride), or regular soap and water should be used to clean the site before blood alcohol collection. Use of an alcohol-containing antiseptic could lead to contamination of the specimen and cause erroneous results. Isopropanol and methanol are types of alcohol. Anything that is a tincture, such as tincture of iodine, contains alcohol.

19. *d.* No food, alcohol, smoking, or chewing gum is allowed throughout the test period. The stimulants in coffee, tea, and cigarettes will alter the values. Even sugarless gum will affect the test results due to the stimulation of the digestive process.

20. *d.* Glycosuria means a condition of having sugar in the urine and is easily measured using a urine dipstick. The

other instruments perform testing on blood samples.

21. *c.* Skin tests involve the intradermal (within the skin) injection of allergenic substance to determine if the patient has come in contact with a specific allergen and developed antibodies against it.

22. *b.* Occult means concealed or hidden. The guaiac test uses chemical means to detect blood that is not visually apparent in a specimen. Occult blood in feces (stool) may signify the presence of colorectal ulcers or cancer.

23. *c.* The timing for collection of specimens of a glucose tolerance test (GTT) begins after the patient finishes the glucose beverage. The phlebotomist will list the schedule of draws from that time forward based on the physician's orders (Fig. 11-3).

24. *c.* The tuberculin test is also called PPD test because of the "purified protein

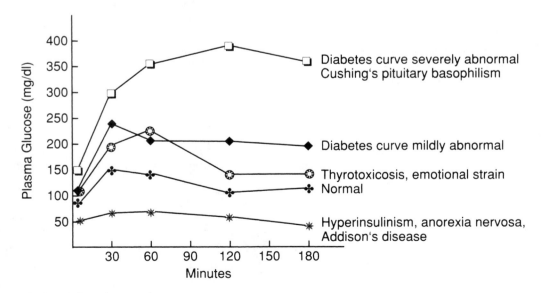

FIGURE 11-3. Glucose tolerance test curves.

derivative" used in testing for tuberculosis. The cocci test is for an infectious fungus disease *Coccidoides immitus*; the histo test is for past or present infection by the fungus *Histoplasma capsulatum*; and the Shick test is for susceptibility to diphtheria.

25. *c.* Drug screen tests may be requested by law enforcement officials for forensic or legal reasons. Special collection protocol requires "chain of custody" procedures providing documentation that the specimen is accounted for at all times.

26. *d.* Interpretation of the test is based on the presence or absence of erythema (redness) and/or induration (hardness). A positive test is when the areas of erythema and induration are 10 mm or greater in diameter.

27. *d.* Therapeutic phlebotomy is performed as a treatment for certain medical conditions, such as polycythemia (overproduction of red cells). It involves the withdrawal of a large volume of blood usually measured by the unit as in blood donation.

28. *c.* The term erythema means redness.

29. *c.* AccuChek, Glucometer, and One-Touch glucose meters all use a test strip for glucose testing. The HemoCue performs the test on venous, arterial, or capillary using a microcuvette rather than a test strip.

30. *d.* Blood T & C is performed to determine the compatibility of blood to be used in a transfusion. If the patient is not identified properly and the specimen labeled exactly, a transfusion can result in death (Fig. 11-4).

31. *b.* It is normal procedure to inflate the blood pressure cuff to 40 mm Hg when performing a BT test. The

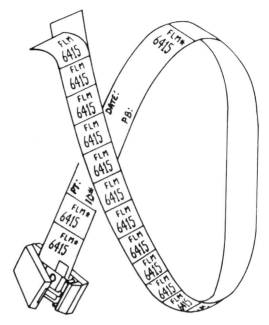

FIGURE 11-4. Typenex bloodbank identification bracelet. (Courtesy of Fenwal Laboratories, a division of Travenol Laboratories, Chicago, IL.)

BT results will be increased by aspirin ingestion, decreased platelet count, and disturbing the plate plug formation with the blotting paper.

32. *b.* A crossmatch normally requires a large, plain (no serum separator gel) red stopper tube because it is important to avoid any additives or reactants in the tube when doing compatibility testing.

33. *d.* During a BT test a blood pressure cuff instead of a tourniquet is used to apply a constant pressure of 40 mm Hg to the arm. A tourniquet is not used because of the inability to standardize the pressure applied. Other equipment used include a special standardized incision device

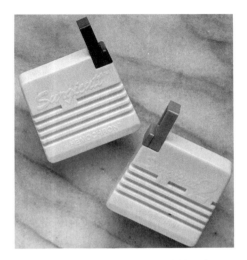

FIGURE 11-5. Surgicutt automated bleeding time device. (Courtesy of International Technidyne, Edison, NJ.)

(Fig. 11-5), a stopwatch, and a butterfly bandage to help close the incision.

34. *b.* Autologous donation is the process by which a person donates blood for his or her own use. This is done for elective surgeries where possibility of transfusion is anticipated.

35. *a.* Skin antisepsis is a very important part of the blood culture collection procedure. Failure to follow sterile technique can introduce skin surface bacteria into the blood culture bottle and interfere with interpretation of results.

36. *a.* The AccuMeter uses fingerstick or venous heparinized whole blood to measure total blood cholesterol by a one-step quantitative visual determination. HemoCue, IRMA, and I-Stat calculate a qualitative value.

37. *c.* Gentamicin, digoxin, and theophylline are all therapeutic drugs, whereas phenylalanine is an amino acid formed from protein.

38. *c.* The hormone first detected in pregnancy testing is human chorionic gonadotropin (HCG). ACTH is adrenocorticotropic hormone, an adrenal hormone. HCT stands for hematocrit. TSH is thyroid-stimulating hormone.

39. *d.* An/aerobic literally means without/air.

40. *c.* The guaiac test detects the presence of occult (hidden) blood in the stool (feces).

41. *c.* The recommended antiseptic for blood culture collection is povidone iodine which when used appropriately comes closest to sterilizing the area.

42. *b.* The blood coagulation process is monitored closely in patients receiving anticoagulants such as heparin and warfarin and for patients undergoing transfusion therapy. Lithium therapy is used in the treatment of depression and has nothing to do with coagulation.

43. *c.* The test procedure involves expediting coagulation time by use of a clot-enhancing substance (activator), such as siliceous earth or celite. The ACT tests the activity of the intrinsic coagulation factors and is used to monitor heparin therapy.

44. *a.* Glucose levels in blood specimens obtained 2 hours after a meal are used as a screening test for carbohydrate metabolism problems. Two-hour postprandial glucose specimens are rarely elevated in normal persons, but may be significantly increased in diabetic patients. The test is also used to monitor insulin therapy.

45. *b.* The BT test detects platelet function disorders by testing platelet plug formation in the capillaries (Fig. 11-6).

46. *c.* A lactose tolerance test is used to determine if a patient lacks the enzyme (mucosal lactase) that is

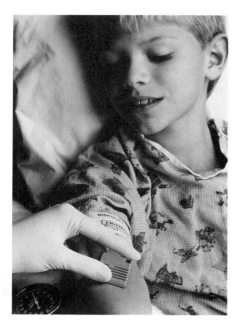

FIGURE 11-6. Bleeding time being performed. (Courtesy of International Technidyne, Edison, NJ.)

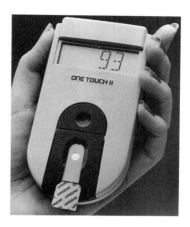

FIGURE 11-7. ONE TOUCH II® Blood Glucose Meter. (Courtesy of LifeScan Inc., Milpitas, CA.)

necessary to convert the milk sugar lactose into glucose and galactose.

47.   *d.*   If a patient undergoing a glucose tolerance test vomits within 30 minutes of drinking the glucose beverage, the patient's physician should be notified to see if the test should be continued. Giving the patient another dose of glucose or noting the vomiting and continuing the test at that point could result in misinterpretation of the results.

48.   *b.*   Reliable glucose monitoring can be done with small hand-held ancillary blood glucose testing (ABGT) analyzers which use whole blood specimens obtained by routine skin puncture. With the ease of collection and analysis, it can be done at the bedside (Fig. 11-7).

49.   *a.*   TDM is used by physicians to manage individual patient drug treatment. It is used to help establish

drug dosages, to maintain dosages at beneficial levels, and to avoid drug toxicity.

50.   *a.*   If a phlebotomist should arrive to collect a 2-hour postprandial specimen and the 2 hours have not elapsed since the patient's meal, the phlebotomist should ask the patient's nurse to verify the correct time to draw the specimen. It is not a good idea to ask the patient what the correct time for collection would be; in most cases, the patient does not know. Nor should the phlebotomist collect the specimen, regardless of the time, because if collected too early, glucose levels may still be elevated and lead to misinterpretation of results.

51.   *b.*   It is not unusual for patients to be on antimicrobial (antibiotic) therapy at the time blood culture specimens are collected. Antimicrobial agents in the patient's blood can inhibit the growth of the microorganisms in the blood culture bottle. In such cases, blood cultures may be collected in a broth vial with an antimicrobial adsorbing resin included.

Arterial Blood Gases

12

REVIEW QUESTIONS

1. The proper angle for femoral ABG puncture is:
   a. 15 degrees
   b. 20 degrees
   c. 54 degrees
   d. 90 degrees

2. An ABG sample must be delivered to the laboratory for analysis within the following time limit:
   a. 5 minutes
   b. 15 minutes
   c. 30 minutes
   d. 60 minutes

3. Which artery is generally the easiest to access during low cardiac output?
   a. brachial
   b. femoral
   c. radial
   d. ulnar

4. The artery of choice for ABGs is:
   a. brachial
   b. femoral
   c. radial
   d. ulnar

5. When performing the Allen test, which artery is released first?

a. brachial
b. femoral
c. radial
d. ulnar

6. What happens to an ABG specimen left at room temperature?
   a. blood cells will continue to consume oxygen
   b. the specimen will hemolyze
   c. carbon dioxide levels will stabilize
   d. all of the above

7. After performing ABGs, check the pulse:
   a. distal to the puncture site
   b. in the ulnar artery
   c. medial to the puncture site
   d. proximal to the puncture site

8. Which of the following is the most common arterial puncture complication even when proper technique is used?
   a. arteriospasm
   b. hematoma
   c. infection
   d. thrombus formation

9. ABGs should be transported:
   a. as soon as possible
   b. after air bubbles have been removed
   c. on ice
   d. all of the above

10. The purpose of the Allen test is to:
    a. check for collateral circulation
    b. determine blood pressure
    c. make certain that you have palpated an artery
    d. see if you need to deaden the nerve

11. After obtaining an ABG, the phlebotomist is unable to maintain pressure on the puncture site for the required amount of time. The site has stopped bleeding; what should she do?
    a. apply a pressure bandage after checking to ensure there is no excessive bleeding
    b. find a nurse to hold the site, giving her explicit instructions
    c. instruct the patient to carefully hold the site
    d. leave the site alone, after checking to ensure there is no excessive bleeding

12. What is the correct equipment to use when collecting an ABG?
    a. butterfly and syringe
    b. heparinized evacuated tube
    c. special plastic syringe
    d. any of the above

13. A disadvantage of using the brachial artery for ABG collection is the fact that it is:
    a. harder to compress
    b. near a large nerve
    c. near the basilic vein
    d. all of the above

14. The most common needle size for radial ABGs is:
    a. 18 gauge
    b. 20 gauge
    c. 22 gauge
    d. 25 gauge

15. To maintain the integrity of the arterial blood sample, the sample should be:
    a. cooled in crushed ice immediately after drawing
    b. kept at room temperature until tested
    c. placed in a heat block and taken to the laboratory as soon as possible
    d. placed in the refrigerator upon arrival in the laboratory

16. Too much anticoagulant in the ABG syringe can cause:
    a. bubbles in the sample
    b. inaccurate results
    c. makes no difference
    d. the blood to clot

17. Which of the following tests requires an arterial specimen?
    a. ammonia
    b. blood cultures
    c. blood gases
    d. glycohemoglobin

18. Which of the following would be a reason for rejecting an ABG specimen?
    a. clotted specimen
    b. improper label
    c. inadequate volume
    d. all of the above

19. What is the *biggest* advantage in choosing a radial artery for ABG collection?
    a. it works best during low cardiac output
    b. it is large and easy to locate
    c. it is easy to compress to stop bleeding
    d. the presence of collateral circulation

20. Which of the following conditions would eliminate the site as a choice for ABG collection?
    a. inflammation
    b. edema
    c. fistula
    d. all of the above

21. Which of the following is the proper procedure if the patient *does not* have collateral circulation?
    a. check the circulation in the other arm
    b. perform ABGs on the radial artery
    c. perform ABGs on the ulnar artery
    d. perform femoral ABGs

22. Heparin is used during ABG procedure to:
    a. ease the pain
    b. increase blood flow
    c. prevent clotting of the blood in the syringe
    d. stabilize oxygen content of the blood

23. The purpose of lidocaine in ABG collection is to:
    a. help dissolve air bubbles
    b. keep the specimen from clotting
    c. numb the site
    d. stabilize the specimen

24. Which of the following *is not* necessary ABG equipment?
    a. 2- to 5-mL syringe
    b. alcohol and betadyne
    c. proper anticoagulant
    d. tourniquet

25. Which of the following should *not* cause erroneous ABG results?
    a. ignoring air bubbles in the specimen
    b. transporting the specimen on ice
    c. processing the specimen after 30 minutes
    d. use of EDTA as the anticoagulant

26. Which patient would be considered to be in a "steady state" as applied to blood gas collection? The patient has:
    a. been on a ventilator for 10 minutes
    b. been breathing room air and sleeping for 30 minutes
    c. just finished eating breakfast
    d. just returned from radiology

27. The proper angle for drawing radial ABGs is:
    a. 15 degrees
    b. 25 degrees
    c. 45 degrees
    d. 90 degrees

28. Which arterial site poses the greatest risk of infection?
    a. brachial
    b. femoral
    c. radial
    d. ulnar

29. The needle length of choice for femoral ABGs is:
    a. 1 inch
    b. 1½ inch
    c. 2 inch
    d. 2½ inch

30. Which of the following is *not* a blood gas component?
    a. P_{CO_2}
    b. pH
    c. P_{O_2}
    d. PO_4

31. Which of the following is the *best* way to tell if a specimen is arterial? As the specimen is collected, the blood:
    a. appears bright cherry red
    b. contains air bubbles

   c. looks dark bluish red in color
   d. pumps into the syringe

32. When collecting ABGs, the latex cube is used to:
   a. cap the syringe during transport
   b. collect air bubbles from the needle
   c. contain the needle while the phlebotomist is holding pressure on the artery
   d. none of the above

33. The proper solution for cleaning an ABG site is:
   a. heparin
   b. lidocaine
   c. povidone iodine
   d. sodium hypochlorite

34. When performing ABGs, direct the needle:
   a. away from the hand and facing the blood flow
   b. direction doesn't matter as long as the bevel is up
   c. perpendicular to the wrist
   d. toward the hand and facing the blood flow

35. A patient who has collateral circulation:
   a. cannot undergo radial blood gas collection
   b. has more than one artery supplying blood to the area
   c. has normal cardiac output
   d. is well ventilated

ANSWERS TO REVIEW QUESTIONS

1. *d.* The angle required for a femoral puncture is 90 degrees due to the location and depth of the artery.

2. *b.* An ABG specimen must be delivered to the laboratory in an ice slurry within 5 to 10 minutes of collection. Time is critical to the integrity of specimen because although cooling the sample slows metabolism, it does not completely stop changes that may affect results.

3. *b.* The femoral artery is large and easily punctured. It is sometimes the only site where arterial sampling is possible, especially on patients with low cardiac output.

4. *c.* The radial artery, located in the thumb side of the wrist (Fig. 12-1) is the first choice and consequently the most common site used for arterial blood gas collection.

5. *c.* In the Allen test (Fig. 12-2), the pressure on the ulnar artery is released first to check for adequate arterial blood flow into the hand. The patient's hand should flush pink within 15 seconds.

6. *a.* If an arterial blood sample is left at room temperature, the blood cells will continue to consume oxygen and use glucose resulting in increased CO_2 and lactic acid levels and a change in pH. Erroneous ABG results will be the outcome.

7. *a.* The pulse distal to the puncture site should be checked after performing the ABG to ensure there is no damage which might occlude the blood flow. If there is no pulse the patient's nurse should be notified immediately so that measures can be taken to restore circulation.

8. *a.* Even when proper technique is used in arterial puncture, complications can occur. The most common complication is arteriospasm, caused by a reflex constriction of the artery muscle when the needle penetrates the artery wall. Hematoma (bruising), thrombus (clot) formation, and infection are most often caused by improper technique. However, infection can result in patients with compromised immune systems even when proper technique is used.

9. *d.* After the needle is withdrawn and any air bubbles are ejected from the specimen, the needle is embedded into a small latex cube and the specimen is placed in crushed ice for delivery to the laboratory for testing.

10. *a.* The Allen test (see Fig. 12-2) is performed to check for collateral circulation which means that the area is supplied with blood from more than one artery. In the event that the artery is damaged during ABG collection, the other artery will maintain blood flow to the hand.

11. *a.* If the phlebotomist cannot apply pressure to an ABG site for the required amount of time, she should check the site for excessive bleeding, swelling, or bruising and clean the povidone iodine from the site. If the bleeding has stopped, the site appears normal and there is a good pulse distal to the site, the phlebotomist can apply a pressure bandage to be removed later by the nurse.

12. *c.* Special glass or plastic 1- to 5-mL syringes (Fig. 12-3) are recommended

text continues on page 184

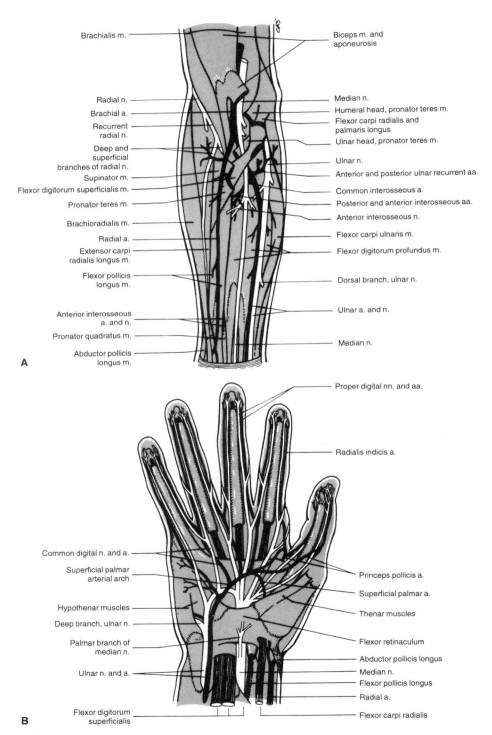

FIGURE 12-1. Arteries of the arm **(A)** and hand **(B).**

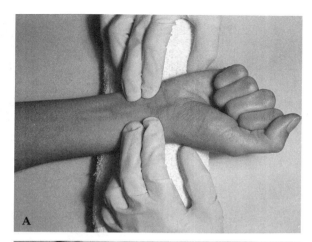

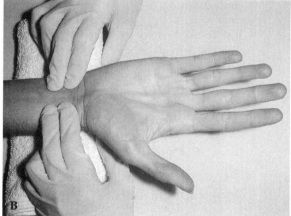

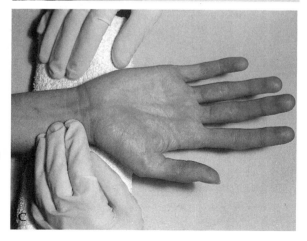

FIGURE 12-2. Allen test. **(A)** Occluding the radial and ulnar arteries by pressing with fingertips while the patient makes a fist. **(B)** Observing a blanched appearance to the hand when opened as both arteries are being pressed. **(C)** Releasing the ulnar artery and checking for the patient's hand to flush with color.

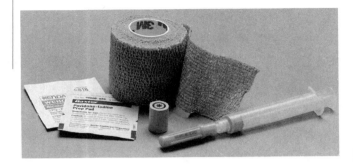

FIGURE 12-3. ABG equipment.

for ABG collection. Heparin-containing syringes are available in special blood gas kits. Using a butterfly to collect a specimen would not be appropriate because the air in the tubing would lead to erroneous results. ABGs cannot be collected using the evacuated tube system.

13. *d.* There are several disadvantages to puncturing the brachial artery: (1) it is deeper than the radial artery making it more difficult to compress after the puncture; and (2) it lies close to the large basilic vein and the median nerve which can be inadvertently punctured during the procedure.

14. *c.* A 22-gauge, 1-inch needle is most commonly used for radial and brachial puncture.

15. *a.* To maintain the integrity of the arterial blood sample, the blood must be cooled in crushed ice immediately after drawing. If the specimen remains at room temperature for more than 5 to 10 minutes, the pH, blood gases, and glucose values will change because of cellular metabolism.

16. *b.* Too much heparin will cause acidosis and therefore, erroneous results.

17. *c.* The primary reason for performing arterial puncture is to obtain blood for evaluation of ABGs.

18. *d.* The laboratory cannot accept any specimen that is improperly labeled. A specimen that does not contain sufficient blood to do the test is referred to as a "short" or "QNS" (quantity not sufficient) specimen. ABGs must be performed on whole blood samples. Even microclots will invalidate test results.

19. *d.* Because it is not uncommon to irritate a vessel when performing an arterial puncture, the biggest advantage of using the radial artery is the presence of collateral circulation. Then if the radial artery were to be inadvertently damaged, the ulnar artery could supply blood to the hand.

20. *d.* Irritation or inflammation of the site and swelling or edema may cause erroneous results. Drawing an ABG from an arm with an AV shunt or fistula because of the merger of a vein an artery will cause inaccurate results.

21. *a.* If the Allen test shows that the patient does not have collateral circulation in one arm, the other arm should be checked before considering the brachial or femoral artery.

22. *c.* The anticoagulant used to prevent the blood from clotting during the ABG procedure is heparin. When it is used

in the right amount it does not alter the blood pH and blood gases values as other anticoagulants might.

23. *c.* Lidocaine is a local anesthetic drug which may be used to numb the arterial puncture site.

24. *d.* Tourniquets are not used when collecting ABGs because the pressure in the arterial system keeps the vessel inflated and the pulse aids the phlebotomist in locating the artery (see Fig. 12-3).

25. *b.* Erroneous ABG results can be caused by ignoring air bubbles in the specimen, not processing the specimen within 30 minutes, and using an anticoagulant other than EDTA. An ABG *should be* transported on ice to slow down metabolism and maintain the integrity of the sample.

26. *b.* A patient's temperature and breathing pattern affect the amount of oxygen and carbon dioxide in the blood. Ideally, a patient should have been in a stable state (no exercise, eating, sectioning, or respiratory changes) for at least 30 minutes before obtaining blood gases.

27. *c.* When doing a radial or brachial puncture, the needle is inserted bevel up into the skin at a 45-degree angle (Fig. 12-4).

28. *b.* The femoral artery (Fig. 12-5) is located superficially in the groin area lateral to the pubis bone. This site poses the greatest risk of infection because of the difficulty in achieving aseptic technique because of the presence of pubic hair.

29. *b.* The needle length of choice for femoral ABGs is 1½ inch because the needle may have to penetrate several layers of subcutaneous tissue as it

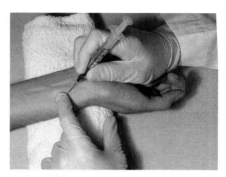

FIGURE 12-4. Performing an arterial puncture.

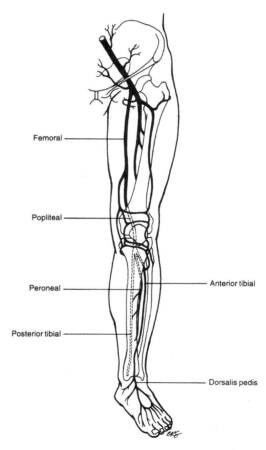

Femoral

Popliteal

Peroneal

Anterior tibial

Posterior tibial

Dorsalis pedis

FIGURE 12-5. Arteries of the leg.

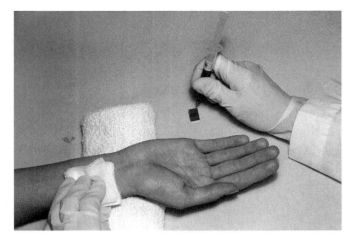

FIGURE 12-6. Embedding the point of the ABG needle in the latex cube while holding pressure over the patient's artery.

goes from the surface of the skin to the femoral artery.

30. *d.* The components measured in the blood gases analysis are: P_{CO_2}, pH, and P_{O_2}. $P0_4$ is the designation for phosphorous and is not a blood gas component.

31. *d.* As the specimen is collected, the blood will pump into the syringe if it is arterial. The color of arterial blood, normally bright cherry red, is not a consistent indicator of a successful arterial puncture because patients with pulmonary conditions do not have oxygen-rich, cherry red arterial blood.

32. *a.* The small latex cube plays an important part in the ABG procedure. Immediately after the needle is withdrawn and any air bubbles are ejected from the specimen, the needle is embedded

into the small latex cube (Fig. 12-6) to prevent contamination of the specimen from room air while being transported.

33. *c.* Povidone iodine or Betadyne is used to clean an ABG site in an effort to minimize the chance of infection. Heparin is the anticoagulant used in the syringe. Lidocaine is an anesthetic used to numb the site before arterial puncture. Sodium hypochlorite (bleach) is a disinfectant used to clean blood spills.

34. *a.* The position of the needle and syringe for ABG collection is away from the hand and facing the blood flow as shown in Figure 12-3.

35. *b.* Collateral circulation means that the patient has both the radial and the ulnar artery supplying blood to the hand.

Nonblood Specimens and Tests

13

REVIEW QUESTIONS

1. Amniotic fluid is obtained from within the:
   a. abdominal cavity
   b. membrane that surrounds a fetus
   c. sac surrounding the heart
   d. space within a joint

2. Semen analysis is performed for the purpose of determining:
   a. bladder function

   b. circumcision candidates
   c. fertility
   d. prostatic cancer

3. What type of specimen is required for a biopsy?
   a. stool
   b. sweat
   c. tissue
   d. urine

4. What is the recommended procedure for collecting a 24-hour urine sample?
   a. collect all the urine voided in any 24-hour period
   b. collect the first morning specimen and all the following specimens except the next morning specimen
   c. start the timing, collect the first morning specimen, and collect all the following specimens including the first specimen the next morning
   d. void the first morning specimen, start the timing, and collect all the following specimens, including the next morning's specimen

5. This fluid is obtained by lumbar puncture?
   a. peritoneal
   b. pleural
   c. spinal
   d. synovial

6. Which of the following tests is handled and analyzed STAT?
   a. CSF
   b. gastric analysis
   c. occult blood
   d. urinalysis (UA)

7. Which of the following fluids comes from the peritoneal cavity?
   a. ascitic fluid
   b. gastric secretion
   c. sputum
   d. synovial fluid

8. Which semen specimen most likely would be rejected for testing? A specimen:
   a. collected in a condom
   b. delivered in a sterile container
   c. kept at 37° C
   d. obtained on site

9. Spinal fluid tests include all of the following *except*:
   a. cell count
   b. glucose
   c. protein
   d. hemoglobin

10. What special information is required when labeling a nonblood specimen?
    a. biohazard warning
    b. ordering physician
    c. special handling needs
    d. specimen source

11. This test requires intravenous administration of histamine or pentagastrin:
    a. gastric analysis
    b. glucose tolerance test (GTT)
    c. epinephrine tolerance test
    d. sweat chloride

12. Which test is used to diagnose cystic fibrosis?
    a. bleeding time
    b. occult blood
    c. semen analysis
    d. sweat chloride

13. Spinal fluid analysis is used in the diagnosis of:
    a. diabetes
    b. meningitis
    c. osteoporosis
    d. renal failure

14. "Clean-catch" urine collection requires:
    a. a sterile container
    b. cleaning the genital area
    c. midstream collection
    d. all of the above

15. Fluid from the lung cavity is called:
    a. pericardial fluid
    b. peritoneal fluid
    c. pleural fluid
    d. synovial fluid

16. Which of the following is the *best* specimen for routine is?
    a. fasting
    b. first voided
    c. random
    d. 24 hour

17. Which test is commonly performed on amniotic fluid?
    a. alkaline phosphatase

b. alpha-fetoprotein
c. disseminated intravascular coagulation
d. lactic dehydrogenase

18. Fluid from joint cavities is called:
    a. pericardial fluid
    b. peritoneal fluid
    c. pleural fluid
    d. synovial fluid

19. Specimens for routine UA that cannot be processed within 2 hours require:
    a. a preservative
    b. recollection
    c. refrigeration
    d. room temperature storage

20. Which statement is *not* true of urine creatinine clearance specimen collection?
    a. a 24-hour specimen is required
    b. a blood creatinine is also collected
    c. refrigeration is preferred
    d. requires a double-voided specimen

21. A refrigerated stool sample would *not* be acceptable for:
    a. culture
    b. fat analysis
    c. occult blood
    d. ova and parasites

22. Gastric fluid does *not* normally contain:
    a. blood
    b. HCL
    c. mucus
    d. pepsin

23. A urine C & S is ordered to check for:
    a. abnormal urine pH
    b. glucose spillage into the urine
    c. presence of UTI
    d. specific gravity

24. Iontophoresis is used in the collection of which type specimen?
    a. semen
    b. sweat
    c. tears
    d. urine

25. What is sputum?
    a. bronchial secretions
    b. gastric fluid
    c. nasal mucus
    d. saliva

26. A midstream "clean-catch" urine specimen is required for a:
    a. 24-hour urine test
    b. GTT
    c. routine UA
    d. urine C & S

27. What can happen to urine components if not processed in a timely fashion?
    a. bacteria multiply
    b. bilirubin breaks down
    c. cellular elements decompose
    d. all of the above

28. Which test requires a 24-hour stool specimen?
    a. Epstein-Barr virus
    b. thyroxine
    c. tuberculosis
    d. urobilinogen

29. A NP culture swab is collected to detect the presence of organisms that cause:
    a. genetic defects
    b. strep throat
    c. UTI
    d. whooping cough

30. Peritoneal fluid comes from the:
    a. abdominal cavity
    b. lung cavity
    c. pericardial sac
    d. spinal cavity

31. What specimen is required for a "rapid strep" test?
    a. blood sample
    b. stool specimen
    c. throat swab
    d. urine specimen

ANSWERS TO REVIEW QUESTIONS

1. *b.* Amniotic fluid is obtained from within the membrane (amniotic sac) that surrounds a fetus in the uterus. A physician obtains the fluid by inserting a needle through the patient's abdominal wall and uterus and into the amniotic sac. Amniotic fluid can be tested to determine gestational age, lung maturity, and genetic defects of the fetus.

2. *c.* Semen analysis is used to assess fertility and also to determine the effectiveness of sterilization following vasectomy.

3. *c.* A biopsy is the excision (removal) of a small piece of living tissue in order to microscopically examine it. Biopsy samples are examined in the histology department.

4. *d.* The recommended procedure for a 24-hour urine collection is as follows: The best time to start the test is in the morning upon waking. Void as usual into the toilet and note the time and date. Collect all urine voided for the next 24-hour period. At the end of the 24-hour period, usually upon rising the following morning, void one last time, adding this specimen to the collection container.

5. *c.* CSF fills the space between the meninges and the spinal cord. A physician obtains CSF through lumbar (spinal) puncture.

6. *a.* CSF must be delivered to the laboratory "STAT" and analysis started immediately. CSF is obtained by a physician, most often through lumbar puncture, and should be handled carefully and quickly so that the specimen is not compromised.

7. *a.* Ascites is a clear, pale straw-colored, serous fluid aspirated from the peritoneal cavity.

8. *a.* Semen specimens should be collected in sterile containers and never in a condom. Condoms often contain spermicide which would invalidate the results.

9. *d.* Common tests performed on CSF include cell counts, glucose, chloride, and total protein. Red blood cells and hemoglobin are not normally found in CSF, except as a contaminant from the aspiration procedure.

10. *d.* As a minimum, nonblood specimens should be labeled with the same identifying information as blood specimens. Most institutions also require information on the source of the specimen. A biohazard warning and special handling information are required when shipping a specimen to another laboratory. Putting the name of the ordering physician on the label is usually optional.

11. *a.* A basal tube gastric analysis involves aspirating gastric secretions following a period of fasting. Afterwards a gastric stimulant, most commonly histamine or pentagastrin, is administered intravenously and several more samples are collected at timed intervals.

12. *d.* A sweat chloride test is used in the diagnosis of cystic fibrosis. Cystic fibrosis is caused by a disorder of the exocrine glands, affecting primarily the lungs, liver, and pancreas. Children with cystic fibrosis have abnormally high levels of chloride in their sweat.

13. *b.* An increased white blood cell count in CSF is most often associated with bacterial or viral meningitis.

14. *d.* "Clean-catch" urine collection ensures that the specimen is free of contaminating matter from the external genital areas. Collection procedures include cleaning the genital area (usually with special towelettes), and collecting the specimen "midstream" into a sterile container (Fig. 13-1).

15. *c.* Pleural fluid is aspirated from the pleural cavity, which surrounds the lungs.

16. *b.* The type of specimen preferred for most urine studies is the first urine voided (passed naturally from the bladder or urinated) in the morning.

17. *b.* Alpha-fetoprotein is an antigen normally present in the human fetus; it is found in amniotic fluid and also maternal serum. Alpha-fetoprotein values differ for each week of gestation. The test is performed to see if the fetus is developing normally.

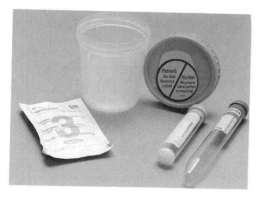

FIGURE 13-1. Becton-Dickinson (Franklin Lakes, NJ) midstream urine collection sampling container and evacuated tubes for transporting and storing urine specimens.

18. *d.* A colorless lubricating fluid aspirated from joint cavities is called synovial fluid.

19. *c.* Specimens for routine UA that cannot be transported or analyzed promptly can be held at room temperature and protected from light for up to 2 hours. Specimens held longer should be refrigerated. Under normal circumstances, specimens for routine UA do not require a preservative. A preservative may be required for certain 24-hour specimens. Any specimens inappropriately handled may need to be recollected.

20. *d.* Creatinine clearance urine specimen collection requires a 24-hour refrigerated specimen and a blood creatinine specimen. It does not involve a double-voided specimen. A double-voided specimen is collected to compare the concentration of an analyte at two separate specific times.

21. *d.* Some stool specimens, especially those for detection of parasites, should be kept at body temperature (37° C). Refrigerating the sample causes the parasites to encyst making it very difficult to identify and diagnose the condition.

22. *a.* Normal gastric fluid is thin and colorless and contains pepsin, hydrochloric acid (HCL), and mucus. Blood should not be present unless there is hemorrhage (bleeding), as in carcinoma or ulceration.

23. *c.* A urine culture and sensitivity may be requested on a patient with symptoms of urinary tract infection (UTI).

24. *b.* During a sweat chloride test a process called iontophoresis is used to stimulate sweat production. Iontophoresis involves transporting the sweat stimulating drug

pilocarpine into the skin by means of electrical stimulation from electrodes placed on the skin.

25. *a.* Sputum is bronchial secretions obtained through deep coughing. Substances produced after a light cough may be saliva or material from the throat, not sputum.

26. *d.* Urine for C & S should be collected in a sterile container following "clean-catch" midstream procedures (see Fig. 13-1).

27. *d.* The components dissolved in the urine sample will begin to decompose if not processed in a timely fashion. The bilirubin in the urine will change to biliverdin; the cellular elements will become unidentifiable and bacteria that are present will quickly multiply.

28. *d.* Urobilinogen testing is sometimes performed on 24-, 48-, or 72-hour

stool specimens. The specimen is collected in a large gallon container similar to a paint can. It must be refrigerated throughout the collection period.

29. *d.* Nasopharyngeal culture swabs are collected to detect the presence of the microorganisms that cause diphtheria, meningitis, pneumonia, and pertussis (whooping cough).

30. *a.* Peritoneal fluid is aspirated from the abdominal cavity.

31. *c.* A "rapid strep" test is used to diagnose streptococcal (strep) infections and is most often performed on a throat swab. The test can be collected and completed in the physician's office for quick diagnosis and start of appropriate therapy.

Quality Assurance and Specimen Handling and Processing

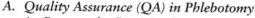

A. Quality Assurance (QA) in Phlebotomy
1. Reasons for Participating
2. QA Defined
3. Identifying QA Indicators
4. Establishing Thresholds and Evaluating Data
5. Quality Control Defined

B. Areas of Phlebotomy Subject to Quality Control
1. Patient Preparation Procedures
2. Specimen Collection Procedures
   a. Identification
   b. Labeling
   c. Technique
   d. Collection Priorities
   e. Continuing Education
3. Documentation
   a. Floor Book
   b. Reference Laboratory Book
   c. Laboratory Procedure Manual
   d. Quality Assurance Forms
      (1) Equipment Check Forms
      (2) Internal Reports

C. Specimen Handling
1. General Guidelines
2. Handling of Routine Specimens
   a. Additive Tube Mixing
   b. Transporting Specimens
      (1) General Guidelines
      (2) Off-Site Transportation Methods
         (a) Packaging
         (b) Labeling
         (c) Temperature Requirements

3. Specimens Requiring Special Handling
   a. Protection From Light
   b. Chilled Specimens
   c. Body Temperature Specimens
4. Time Constraints for Specimen Delivery
5. Exceptions to the Preceding Guidelines

D. Specimen Processing
1. Occupational Safety and Health Administration (OSHA) Regulations
2. Central Processing (Triage)
   a. Receiving
      (1) Validating
         (a) Principle
         (b) Criteria for Specimen Rejection
      (2) Prioritizing
      (3) Accessioning
   b. Specimen Preparation
      (1) Nonblood Specimens
      (2) Whole Blood
      (3) Plasma
      (4) Serum
   c. Special Precautions for Handling Specimens
   d. Centrifugation
      (1) Specimen Preparation
      (2) Centrifuge Operation
   e. Stopper Removal
   f. Aliquot Preparation
   g. Routing
      (1) Dispatching to Testing Area
   h. Referencing
   i. Specimen Storage

REVIEW QUESTIONS

1. Which of the following actions will compromise the quality of the specimen?
   a. drawing electrolytes in an amber tube
   b. mixing a serum separator tube
   c. partially filling a liquid EDTA tube
   d. placing a cold agglutinin in a heat block

2. Which of the following tests would be most affected by contamination from a drop of perspiration?
   a. blood urea nitrogen (BUN)
   b. complete blood count (CBC)
   c. electrolytes
   d. glucose

3. What protective equipment is required when processing specimens?
   a. face shield
   b. fluid-resistant apron
   c. gloves
   d. all of the above

4. Which of the following is *not* a principle of total quality management?
   a. constant improvement
   b. customer satisfaction
   c. employee participation
   d. reduction in staff

5. What special handling does a bilirubin specimen require?
   a. protection from light
   b. transport at body temperature
   c. transport on ice
   d. none of the above

6. You insert a needle into the patient's arm and the patient moves, knocking the needle out. On the second attempt you miss the vein. What do you do next?
   a. ask another phlebotomist to draw the patient
   b. ask the nurse to cancel the request
   c. attempt to draw the patient again
   d. have the nurse draw the specimen from an arterial line

7. Examples of quality control are all of the following *except*:
   a. check expiration dates of evacuated tubes
   b. document maintenance on centrifuge
   c. record refrigerator temperature daily
   d. fill out your time sheet daily

8. To avoid airborne infection while processing specimens:
   a. apply brake when stopping the centrifuge
   b. "pop" the stoppers when opening tubes
   c. pour specimens into aliquot tubes
   d. use a stopper remover or cover the stopper with gauze when removing tube stoppers

9. Chilling will affect quality of test results for which of the following analytes?
   a. ammonia
   b. lactic acid
   c. potassium
   d. renin

10. When the threshold value of a clinical indicator of QA is exceeded and a problem is identified:
    a. a corrective action plan is implemented
    b. an incident report must be filed
    c. patient specimens must always be redrawn
    d. patient's physicians must be notified

11. A nonadditive specimen is spun in a centrifuge to obtain:
    a. buffy coat
    b. plasma
    c. serum
    d. whole blood

12. According to the National Committee for Clinical Laboratory Standards (NCCLS), the maximum time limit for separating serum or plasma from cells is;
    a. 15 minutes
    b. 30 minutes

    c. 1 hour

    d. 2 hours

13. A glucose specimen drawn in a sodium fluoride tube is stable at room temperature for:

    a. 2 hours

    b. 6 hours

    c. 12 hours

    d. 24 hours

14. Which is of the following does *not* represent a QA procedure?

    a. centrifuging specimens that require chilling in a temperature-controlled centrifuge

    b. centrifuging specimens with the tube stoppers off

    c. covering light-sensitive specimens with foil

    d. transporting cold agglutinin specimens in a heat block

15. Gloves with calcium-containing powder are:

    a. a likely source of specimen contamination

    b. ideal for collecting skin puncture specimens

    c. ideal for use in specimen processing

    d. very difficult to put on

16. A phlebotomy collection procedure manual contains:

    a. patient accession numbers

    b. incident reports

    c. detailed procedures for each test performed

    d. phlebotomist performance evaluations

17. The agency that requires health care organizations to have a QA program in place in order to be accredited is:

    a. College of American Pathologists (CAP)

    b. Joint Committee for Accrediting Healthcare Organizations (JCAHO)

    c. NCCLS

    d. OSHA

18. Which of the following conditions would *not* be a reason to reject a specimen for analysis?

    a. a bilirubin specimen is icteric

    b. a CBC specimen has clots in it

    c. an electrolyte specimen is hemolyzed

    d. a fasting glucose specimen is lipemic

19. A specimen was mislabeled on the floor. You are required to fill out an incident report form. What information would you *not* include?

    a. description of the consequence

    b. details of the correction action taken

    c. explanation of the problem

    d. suggestion for new guidelines

20. An aliquot is a:

    a. filter used to separate serum from cells

    b. portion of a specimen being tested

    c. substance being tested

    d. tube used to balance the centrifuge

21. You have already drawn a serum potassium level on a patient. The physician asks you to add a vitamin B_{12} level to the order as you leave the patient's room. What should you do?

    a. apologize to the patient and draw another tube

    b. come back later to draw the B_{12}

    c. cover the specimen with foil and submit for both tests

    d. divide the sample into two tubes

22. A courier delivers an unlabeled STAT specimen from the emergency department drawn by a physician. Laboratory policy prohibits you from accepting an unlabeled specimen. How do you handle the situation?

    a. allow the courier to label the specimen

    b. keep the specimen until the physician comes to label it

    c. label the specimen with information provided over the phone

    d. refuse to accept the specimen and send it back with the courier

23. Minimum precentrifugation time for specimens drawn in serum separator tubes is:
    a. 5 minutes
    b. 10 minutes
    c. 15 minutes
    d. 30 minutes

24. An example of a QA indicator is:
    a. all phlebotomists will follow universal precautions
    b. laboratory personnel will not wear laboratory coats when on break
    c. no eating, drinking, or smoking are allowed in laboratory work areas
    d. the contamination rate for blood cultures will not exceed the national contamination rate

25. Which of the following specimens will be automatically rejected if the tube is *not* filled until the vacuum is exhausted?
    a. CBC
    b. electrolytes
    c. glucose
    d. prothrombin time

26. Vigorous tube mixing can cause hemolysis which will affect the test results of all of the following analytes *except*:
    a. hemoglobin
    b. lactic dehydrogenase
    c. magnesium
    d. potassium

27. Your hospital uses barcode specimen labels. What information must be added to the label whenever a specimen is collected?
    a. date of birth
    b. medical record number
    c. patient's full name
    d. phlebotomist's identification

28. Which specimen needs to be transported on ice?
    a. ammonia
    b. bilirubin
    c. CBC
    d. cold agglutinins

29. What laboratory reference describes in detail the steps to follow for specimen collection?
    a. OSHA Safety Manual
    b. Policy Guidelines
    c. Quality Control Procedures
    d. Procedure Manual/Floor Book

30. Which statement describes proper centrifuge operation?
    a. "balance" specimens by placing tubes of equal size and volume opposite one another
    b. centrifuge serum specimens before they have a chance to clot
    c. never centrifuge serum specimens in the same centrifuge with plasma specimens
    d. remove tube stoppers before placing specimens in the centrifuge

31. You are the only phlebotomist in an outpatient drawing center. A physician orders a test that you are not familiar with. What is the most appropriate action to take?
    a. call the physician's office for assistance
    b. draw both a serum and a plasma sample
    c. refer to the user manual for instruction
    d. send the patient to another drawing center

32. How should a cryofibrinogen specimen be transported?
    a. at room temperature
    b. in a 37°C heat block
    c. on ice
    d. protected from light

33. Which chemistry test requires that the serum be separated from the cells within 30 minutes?
    a. calcium
    b. chloride
    c. phosphorous
    d. potassium

34. You are the only phlebotomist on duty. All of the following tests have been ordered for 1600 on different patients. Which specimen, if drawn late, could be most detrimental to the patient's therapy?
    a. 2 hour postprandial (PP)
    b. blood culture
    c. cardiac enzymes
    d. tobramycin level

35. Some test specimens require immediate cooling in an ice and water slurry in order to:
    a. prevent activation of cold agglutinin
    b. prevent clotting
    c. separate serum more completely
    d. slow metabolic processes

ANSWERS TO REVIEW QUESTIONS

1. *c.* The amount of additive in a collection tube is designed to maintain a specific ratio with the amount of blood that would normally fill the tube until the vacuum is exhausted. Although a partially filled EDTA tube may be accepted for testing, results will not be as accurate as they would be if the tube were filled.

2. *c.* Perspiration or sweat contains sodium chloride. Sodium and chloride are part of an electrolyte determination.

3. *d.* OSHA regulations require the wearing of protective equipment when processing specimens. Protective equipment includes gloves, fully buttoned fluid-resistant laboratory coats or aprons, and protective face gear such as masks and goggles with side shields or chin-length face shields.

4. *d.* Total quality management involves four principles: customer satisfaction, constant improvement, employee participation, and orientation to the process. Reduction in staff is not a part of total quality management although it may be a result.

5. *a.* Some test components are broken down in the presence of light, causing falsely decreased values. The most common of these is bilirubin.

6. *b.* A phlebotomist is allowed to make two attempts when obtaining a specimen. If the second attempt is unsuccessful, the phlebotomist should *not* try a third time. Another phlebotomist should take over.

7. *d.* Quality control is a component of a QA program. Phlebotomy quality control involves checking all of the operational procedures to make certain they are performed correctly, such as checking expiration dates, documenting centrifuge maintenance, and recording refrigerator temperatures. Filling out your time sheet is important, but is not considered a quality control procedure.

8. *d.* Airborne infection could result from breathing an infectious aerosol during specimen processing. Using a stopper remover or covering the stopper with a gauze 4 x 4 when removing stoppers will help prevent contamination from aerosols. Other ways to avoid aerosol formation include: *never* apply the break to stop a centrifuge, *do not* "pop" or use a thumb roll motion to remove tube stoppers, and *never* pour specimens into aliquot tubes, use transfer pipettes instead.

9. *c.* Some specimens such as ammonia, lactic acid, and renin require chilling. Other specimens, such as potassium, are adversely affected by chilling, especially if parts of the specimen freeze. Freezing will cause hemolysis and consequently increase plasma potassium levels.

10. *a.* If the threshold of an indicator is exceeded, data are collected and organized to see if there is a problem. If a problem is identified, a corrective action plan is established and implemented.

11. *c.* Specimens for tests requiring serum must be centrifuged. A specimen that has been collected without an additive or anticoagulant will yield serum when centrifuged (Fig. 14-1).

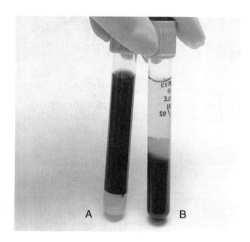

FIGURE 14-1. Hemogard SSTs: **(A)** prior to being centrifuged; **(B)** after being centrifuged.

12. *d.* Guidelines recommended by NCCLS document H18-A set the maximum time limit for separating serum and plasma from the cells at 2 hours from time of collection. Less time is recommended for certain specimens, particularly potassium and cortisol specimens.

13. *d.* According to NCCLS standards, specimens for glucose determination drawn in sodium fluoride tubes are stable for 24 hours at room temperature and up to 48 hours when refrigerated at 2° C to 8° C.

14. *b.* Specimens should be centrifuged with the stoppers on to prevent contamination, evaporation, changes in pH, and aerosol formation.

15. *a.* Gloves must be worn when collecting blood or processing specimens, and powdered gloves are sometimes easier to put on; but powder from gloves can contaminate specimens. Contamination can occur during collection (especially true for skin puncture specimens) or during processing and testing. Some gloves contain calcium powder which could contaminate specimens for calcium determinations and lead to erroneous results.

16. *c.* The phlebotomy collection procedural manual states in detail the step-by-step process for obtaining each laboratory sample.

17. *b.* The JCAHO requires that health care facilities participate in a QA program.

18. *a.* Criteria for specimen rejection include all of the following: a hemolyzed electrolyte specimen, a CBC with clots, and a lipemic specimen for fasting glucose. An icteric specimen is an abnormal dark yellow color caused by jaundice of the patient. The term jaundice is used to describe the yellowness of skin, whites of the eyes, mucous membranes, and body fluids caused by the presence of bile pigments resulting from excess bilirubin in the blood. It is therefore not unusual for a bilirubin specimen to be icteric.

19. *d.* An incident report form (Fig. 14-2) must be filled out when a problem such as a mislabeled specimen occurs. Information on the form must identify the problem, state the consequence, and describe the corrective action. New guidelines are sometimes implemented as a result of an incident, but are not included on the incident report form.

20. *b.* An aliquot is a portion of the specimen used for testing. After centrifugation, the serum or plasma used for testing is placed in labeled tubes called aliquot tubes. If more than one test is to be performed on a single specimen, a portion of the specimen is sometimes placed into several aliquot tubes; especially if different areas of the laboratory perform the various tests ordered.

LINCOLN

EMPLOYEE ACTION RECORD

EMPLOYEE NAME DEPARTMENT DATE

THIS FORM IS USED TO DOCUMENT DISCUSSION CONCERNING A COMMENDATION OR ACTION TAKEN TO IMPROVE INAPPROPRIATE PERFORMANCE BY AN EMPLOYEE. THE INFORMATION CONTAINED ON THIS FORM WILL BE INCLUDED IN THE EMPLOYEE'S PERSONNEL FILE.

( ) COMMENDATION ( ) CORRECTIVE ACTION ( ) OTHER

I. DESCRIBE ISSUE OR INCIDENT (PROVIDE DATES AND DETAILS):

II. PROVIDE SPECIFIC INFORMATION DISCUSSED WITH THE EMPLOYEE REGARDING SECTION I.:

III. PROVIDE THE AGREED-UPON PLAN FOR TAKING CORRECTIVE ACTION, IF APPLICABLE (INCLUDE THE DATE FOR FOLLOW-UP AND NEXT ACTION TO BE TAKEN, IF NECESSARY):

IV. EMPLOYEE COMMENTS:

(ATTACH ADDITIONAL SHEETS IF NECESSARY)

DEPARTMENT MANAGER DATE

EMPLOYEE (SIGNATURE DOES NOT NECESSARILY INDICATE AGREEMENT.) DATE

VICE PRESIDENT DATE

WHITE COPY: HUMAN RESOURCES YELLOW COPY: DIRECTOR PINK COPY: EMPLOYEE

JCL: 04/91 N-115

FIGURE 14-2. Incident form. (Courtesy of John C. Lincoln Hospital, Phoenix, AZ.)

21. *c.* A B_{12} level is also performed on serum. Usually several tests can be performed on the amount of serum collected in a single tube. The best thing to do is immediately wrap the tube in aluminum foil (because light breaks down B_{12}) and submit the specimen for both tests. Light protection will not change the potassium values.

22. *d.* Labeling must be exact. Even a STAT blood sample from the emergency department cannot be accepted if unlabeled. The person who obtains the specimen should be the one who labels it.

23. *c.* Complete clotting or precentrifugation time normally takes around 30 to 45 minutes at room temperature. Specimens drawn in serum separator tubes and other tubes containing clot-activating glass particles usually clot within 15 minutes.

24. *d.* Answers a, b, and c are safety rules. QA indicators are not considered rules but are statements that serve as monitors for all aspects of patient care. By setting a limit or threshold value, they serve as initiators of action plans (Fig. 14-3).

25. *d.* Prothrombin time and most other coagulation specimens collected in a light-blue sodium citrate tube will be rejected for analysis by the laboratory if the tube contains less than 90% of the normal fill. Accurate test results depend on a critical ratio of anticoagulant to blood resulting in a 1:10 dilution. If the dilution is less because of inadequate volume of blood, the results will be falsely elevated.

26. *a.* Potassium, magnesium, and certain enzyme tests, like lactate dehydrogenase, cannot be performed on hemolyzed specimens. A hemoglobin test would not be affected by hemolysis because most methods for determining hemoglobin concentrations lyse the red cells and release the hemoglobin in order to measure it.

27. *d.* Barcode labels (Fig. 14-4) used in specimen collection contain the patient's name, identification number, date, type of specimen, amount, and accession number. The information that must be added is the phlebotomist's identification and time the specimen was collected.

28. *a.* Chilling the specimen keeps the analytes that are being measured as gas, such as ammonia, from escaping into the air in the tube and being lost to the atmosphere as soon as the stopper is removed. Another example of specimens requiring chilling for the same reason is blood gases.

29. *d.* The "laboratory procedure manual" is a reference book that describes in detail the step-by-step process for specimen collection and other procedures performed in the laboratory. A safety manual only contains information on safety issues. A policy manual details management issues, not test collection information. A quality control manual contains procedures and data for the quality control program.

30. *a.* It is imperative that equal size tubes with equal volume of specimen be placed opposite one another or "balanced" in the centrifuge

QUALITY ASSESSMENT AND IMPROVEMENT TRACKING
CONFIDENTIAL A.R.S. 36-445

STANDARD OF CARE/SERVICE: _____

DEPARTMENTS/POPULATION: LABORATORY-MICROBIOLOGY/ALL PATIENTS
DATA SOURCE(S): CULTURE WORKCARDS
DATA COLLECTOR: P. BABINA

IMPORTANT ASPECT OF CARE/SERVICE: LAB SVCS/BLOOD COLLECTION
FREQUENCY REVIEW: 3 MONTHS 100% SAMPLE
METHODOLOGY: RETROSPECITVE
SIGNATURES:
TYPE: OUTCOME
DIRECTOR:
PERSON RESPONSIBLE FOR:
MEDICAL DIRECTOR:
DATA ORGANIZATION: P. BABINA
VICE PRESIDENT/ADMINISTRATOR:
ACTION PLAN: J. BENSON
FOLLOW-UP: J. BENSON
DATE MONITOR BEGAN: 1990
FOLLOW-UP: 3RD QTR.

INDICATORS		THRESHOLD			CRITICAL ANALYSIS/ EVALUATION	ACTION PLAN
		EXP.	ACT.	PREV.		
Blood culture contami-nation rate will not exceed 3% from three groups of drawing per-sonnel.		3%			N= 1385 Patient Centered Care draws: Nur-sing line draws are out of compliance but show improvement from January to March.	A communication has gone out to Nursing reminding to follow esta-blished protocols for drawing. Microbiology has implemented new protocol disallowing a line draw unless two consecutive venipunctures have failed or protocol is over-ridden by physician order. PCC tecs have been reinserviced on proper technique.
LAB	JAN	3%	1.1%			
	FEB		1.8%			
	MAR		1.7%			
PCC	JAN	3%	5.6%			
	FEB		4.8%			
	MAR		3.2%			
LINE DRAWS	JAN	3%	5.6%			
	FEB		7.9%			
	MAR		0.0%			

QICONFID

FIGURE 14-3. TQM form.

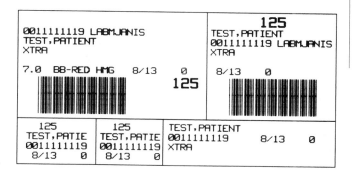

FIGURE 14-4. Barcode label.

(Fig. 14-5). An unbalanced centrifuge may break specimen tubes, ruin the specimen, and cause the contents to form aerosols.

31. *c.* Every drawing center is supplied with a "user manual" from the laboratory to assist the phlebotomist in obtaining an acceptable specimen. The user manual (Fig. 14-6) describes preparation of the patient and special instructions for specimen collection.

32. *b.* Some specimens need to be transported at or near body temperature of 37° C. Two examples are specimens for cold agglutinins and cryofibrinogen. Specimens that need to be kept warm should be transported in a 37° C heat block.

33. *d.* Potassium specimens must be separated from the cells within 30 minutes to prevent hemolysis which will falsely increase the test results.

34. *d.* Collecting a tobramycin level is considered therapeutic drug monitoring. The specimen must be drawn when ordered to allow the pharmacist to accurately calculate how much of the potent drug should administered. If the specimen is drawn late, it can affect the calculation and dosage which could be detrimental to the therapy and well-being of the patient. NOTE: If a therapeutic drug monitoring specimen must be collected at a time other than requested, the *exact* time of draw must be written on the specimen.

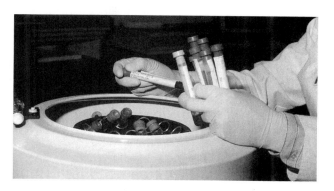

FIGURE 14-5. Specimen processor loading a centrifuge.

HEMATOLOGY

TEST	TEST VOLUME	VACUTAINER COLOR (TOP)	NORMAL VALUES	NOTES
APT test	1 mL feces or gastric fluid	Plastic container	Negative	Suitable for grossly bloody specimens only
Acid hemolysin	0.4 mL (RBC) 2.5 mL serum	Lavender and red (non-Corvac)	0%–5%	
Acid phosphatase stain	3 mL blood	Green		
Acid phosphatase w/tartrate stain (TRAP)	3 mL blood	Green		
Alpha naphthol butyrate stain (nonspecific esterase)	3 mL blood	Green		
Blood smear— differential	.03 mL blood	Lavender or fingerstick	See individual tests	See page 27
Body fluid HCT	1 mL	Fluid		
Bone marrow				Schedule in advance (4-6281)
Coulter count	1 mL blood	Lavender or lavender microtainer	See page 27	Includes WBC, RBC, HGB, HCT, MCV, MCH, MCHC
Differential	1 mL blood	Lavender		See page 28
Eosinophil count	0.5 mL blood	Lavender	150–350 /uL	See page 28
Epinephrine/ endotoxin stimulation test				Schedule in advance (4-6281). Consultation form required
Fetal hemoglobin (APT) (qualitative)	1 mL feces or gastric fluid	Red Non-Corvac or plastic container	Negative	Suitable for grossly bloody specimens only

FIGURE 14-6. User manual. (Courtesy of University Medical Center, Tucson, AZ.)

35. **d.** Certain metabolic processes continue even after the blood leaves the body. Chilling the specimen slows down this process. Specimens requiring chilling should be completely immersed in a slurry of crushed ice and water. Examples of specimens that require chilling are arterial blood gases and ammonia.

Communication and Computers

15

REVIEW QUESTIONS

1. Personal "zone of comfort" is a radius of:
   a. 1 to 18 inches
   b. ½ to 4 feet
   c. 4 to 12 feet
   d. over 12 feet

2. Random access memory (RAM):
   a. can be lost when the computer is turned off
   b. is called firmware
   c. is permanent memory installed by the manufacturer
   d. tells the computer how to begin operations requested by the user

3. Computer peripherals include all of the following *except*:
   a. barcode reader
   b. joystick
   c. modem
   d. central processing unit (CPU)

4. Which of the following is an example of a barrier to effective communication with a patient? The patient:
   a. does not speak English
   b. is a child
   c. is emotionally upset
   d. all of the above

5. Which of the following is an example of a confirming response to a patient?
   a. "I do not know what you mean"
   b. "I have no idea how long it will take"
   c. "I understand how you must be feeling"
   d. "I'm on a tight schedule right now"

6. The laboratory has a computerized LIMS. Once a specimen has been collected by a phlebotomist and returned to the laboratory, what occurs next?
   a. collection labels are printed
   b. collection list is generated
   c. patient information is entered into the system
   d. samples collected are verified

7. The display of options from which a computer user may choose after logging on is called the:
   a. menu
   b. RAM
   c. read only memory (ROM)
   d. CPU

8. Which of the following is an example of negative kinesics?
   a. eye contact
   b. frowning
   c. good grooming
   d. smiling

9. Computer mnemonics are:
   a. accession numbers
   b. hardware
   c. memory aiding codes
   d. tech codes

10. Which of the following is *not* a function of the CPU of a computer?
    a. instructs the computer how to begin operations requested by the user
    b. oversees the completion of tasks required by the operator
    c. performs mathematical processes and logical comparisons of input data
    d. provides the visible display of information being processed

11. Computer input can come from a:
    a. barcode scanner
    b. keyboard
    c. light pen
    d. all of the above

12. Which of the following is *not* part of communicating a professional appearance:
    a. a clean pressed laboratory coat
    b. long hair pulled back
    c. short clean fingernails
    d. wearing strong cologne

13. A computer password:
    a. allows access to the computer
    b. identifies the person using the computer

c. is confidential

d. all of the above

14. Kinesics is the study of:
    a. body language
    b. concepts of control
    c. concepts of space
    d. facial expressions

15. Which of the following examples is a good way to earn a patient's trust?
    a. act knowledgeable
    b. convey sincerity
    c. look professional
    d. all of the above

16. Personal computers are also called:
    a. microcomputers
    b. mainframe computers
    c. minicomputers
    d. supercomputers

17. Which of the following is *not* proper telephone protocol?
    a. answer the phone promptly
    b. clarify and record information
    c. hang up on angry callers
    d. prioritize callers, if necessary

18. A computer outputs information by means of a:
    a. cathode rat tube (CRT)
    b. modem
    c. printer
    d. all of the above

19. Which of the following is an example of proxemics?
    a. eye contact
    b. facial expression
    c. personal hygiene
    d. zone of comfort

20. Which of the following is *not* a recognized basic element of health care communication?
    a. confirmation
    b. control
    c. distrust
    d. empathy

21. A computer terminal is the:
    a. CRT where information is displayed
    b. computer work station composed of a keyboard and CRT as a minimum
    c. end of the electrical cord that plugs into the computer
    d. none of the above

22. A computer that is "on line" is:
    a. being repaired
    b. connected to other computers
    c. hooked to a modem
    d. operational

23. The *best* way to handle a difficult or "bad" patient is:
    a. help the patient to feel in control of the situation
    b. refuse to collect a specimen from him or her
    c. speak sharply to the patient to show that you are in control of the situation
    d. threaten to report the patient to his or her doctor

24. A person who is computer literate can:
    a. adapt to changes that computers are making on quality of life
    b. perform basic operations to complete required tasks
    c. understand the basic components and operations of a computer
    d. all of the above

25. Computer software is:
    a. coded instructions required to process data
    b. equipment used to process data
    c. peripheral equipment used to input data
    d. permanent secondary storage equipment

26. The flashing indicator on the computer screen that indicates the starting point of your input is called the:
    a. CD
    b. cursor
    c. joystick
    d. LIMS

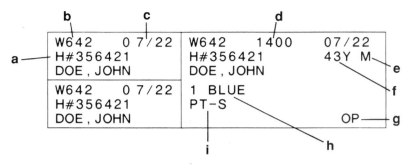

FIGURE 15-1. Computer label.

27. The unit that displays the text as it is entered in a computer is called the:
  a. CRT
  b. ROM
  c. RAM
  d. CD

28. What is the average speaking rate of a normal adult?
  a. 75 to 100 words per minute
  b. 125 to 150 words per minute
  c. 250 to 350 words per minute
  d. 500 to 600 words per minute

29. Proxemics is the study of an individual's:
  a. body language
  b. concept of space
  c. facial expressions
  d. verbal communication

30. Which of the following situations allows the patient to feel in control?
  a. agreeing with the patient that it is his right to refuse to have a blood specimen drawn
  b. informing the patient that you are going to draw a blood sample
  c. insisting that the patient cooperate and let you draw blood

  d. telling the patient not to eat or drink anything during a test

31. Which of the following is used by the laboratory to identify a specimen throughout the testing process?
  a. assession number
  b. hospital number
  c. mnemonic code
  d. tech code

32. In computer language "hard copy" is:
  a. data printed on paper
  b. information displayed on the CRT
  c. information stored on the hard drive
  d. all of the above

For questions 33 to 35 use the choices indicated by the arrows in Figure 15-1 (Figure 16-2 from Phlebotomy Essentials).

33. What letter signifies the time the specimen is to be collected?

34. What letter indicates the type of specimen required?

35. What represents the patient's identification number?

ANSWERS TO REVIEW QUESTIONS

1. *b.* The "zone of comfort" varies with each individual depending largely on how well the intruder is known and other circumstances surrounding the intrusion. For the average individual, intimate distance is a radius of 1 to 18 inches, personal distance is ½ to 4 feet, social distance is 4 to 12 feet, and public distance is a radius of more than 12 feet.

2. *a.* Memory is one of three elements of the CPU. Memory comes in two forms: RAM which provides temporary storage of information that can be lost if computer is turned off; and ROM which is permanent memory installed by the manufacturer that instructs the user how to begin computer operations selected. ROM is sometimes called "firmware" because it has elements of hardware and software.

3. *d.* The CPU is the control unit of the computer that manages and oversees the completion of each task required by the operator. Computer peripherals include all the equipment, other than the CPU, used to input or output information.

4. *d.* All of the above can be barriers to communication and require special communication techniques for effective exchange of information to occur.

5. *c.* Confirming responses help a patient feel recognized as an individual and not a number. "I understand how you must be feeling" is a response that communicates an effort on your part to view the patient as an individual and empathize with his or her situation.

6. *d.* Upon returning from the floor the first thing the phlebotomist must do is verify the specimen so that the nurses on the floor know that the specimen has been collected and no one else will attempt to collect the specimen. Patient information is entered into the system and labels and lists are generated before the specimen is collected.

7. *a.* After logging on, a computer user will see a display of options from which to choose. This display is called the menu.

8. *b.* Frowning is an example of negative kinesics or body language.

9. *c.* Computer mnemonics are memory-aiding codes generally in the form of abbreviations, used to access programs, enter and identify data used or generated by the computer, and perform many other computer functions.

10. *d.* The visible display of information being processed is a function of the CRT, not the CPU.

11. *d.* There are a number of ways to input information to a computer. The most common is a keyboard; but other methods include light pens and barcode readers.

12. *d.* A neat clean appearance plays a big part in presenting a professional image. A clean pressed laboratory coat, short clean fingernails, and long hair pulled back contribute to presenting a professional image. Wearing strong cologne is offensive to some people, especially those who are ill or allergic to perfume, and may interfere with their perceiving the individual who wears it as being professional.

13. *d.* Computer passwords are confidential code words used for security purposes

to allow access as well as identify individuals using a computer system.

14. *a.* Nonverbal communication is called kinesics, the study of body motion or language, such as facial expression, gestures, and eye contact. Body language plays a major role in communication because it is constant and more reliable in interpreting the speaker's true meaning than verbal communication.

15. *d.* Acting knowledgeable, conveying sincerity, and presenting a professional appearance are all part of presenting a professional image that earns a patient's confidence or trust.

16. *a.* Computers can be classified by size. A personal computer is considered a microcomputer, the smallest size classification of computer.

17. *c.* Hanging up on an angry caller does nothing to diffuse the situation and may make it worse. Confirming responses are more apt to calm the caller and allow the problem or situation to be resolved.

18. *d.* Output involves the return of processed information to the user or to someone in another location.

A computer can output information by several means including CRT, printer, or modem.

19. *d.* "Zone of comfort" is an example of proxemics. "Zone of comfort" is a phrase used to describe the invisible "bubble" or range of personal territory that surrounds each of us. When another individual enters this personal territory, we may feel threatened.

20. *c.* Communication between the health professional and the patient is complicated and involves the basic elements of empathy, control, and confirmation. Distrust plays a part in health care communication, but is not one of the basic elements.

21. *b.* As a minimum a computer terminal (Fig. 15-2) consists of a monitor (CRT) and keyboard, which are the essential peripherals for using minicomputers, mainframes, and supercomputers.

22. *d.* When a system is live or operational it is said to be "on line." A computer that is not operational because it is in need of repair is said to be "down." A computer that is "networked" is hooked to other

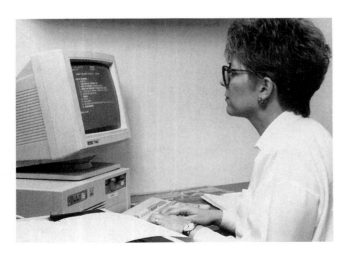

FIGURE 15-2. Health care worker at a microcomputer workstation.

computers. When a computer is hooked to a modem or other peripheral equipment it is said to be "interfaced" with the equipment.

23. *a.* A hospital is one of the few places where an individual gives up control over most of the personal tasks he or she normally performs. Because of this loss of control the patient may respond by getting angry and then is characterized as a "bad" patient.

24. *d.* Computers are becoming commonplace in all walks of life making it essential for more and more workers to become "computer literate" in order to compete successfully in the job market. An individual is generally considered to be computer literate if he or she understands the basic components and functions of a computer, can perform basic computer operations, and is willing to adapt to changes that computers are making on quality of life.

25. *a.* Computer software is the programming or coded instructions needed to control the hardware and process data. There are two types of software. Systems software that controls the normal operation of the computer and applications software which are special programs that perform specific tasks required by the user.

26. *b.* The cursor is a flashing indicator on the screen that indicates where you will start inputting data.

27. *a.* The CRT or monitor is the unit of a computer that displays the text.

28. *b.* The average speaking rate of an adult is 125 to 150 words a minute. Because the average person absorbs verbal messages at 500 to 600 words a minute (which is around five times the speaking rate), the listener must make an effort to stay actively involved in what the speaker is saying to communicate effectively.

29. *b.* Proxemics is the study of an individual's concept and use of space. To better relate to the patient in a health care setting it is important to understand this subtle part of nonverbal communication.

30. *a.* Feeling in control is essential to a patient's well-being. Informing, insisting, and telling are all actions that may cause the patient to feel as if he or she has no control over the situation. Allowing the patient the right to either agree to or refuse a procedure allows the patient to exercise control over the situation and generally makes for a more agreeable patient.

31. *a.* Unlike the hospital number which is used by all departments to identify the patient, the laboratory uses an accession number to identify the specimen. This number is generated by the LIMS when the specimen request is entered into the computer and is unique to that particular specimen. Mnemonic codes are laboratory abbreviations. A tech code is an abbreviation that is unique to the user of the LIMS.

32. *a.* When computer data are printed on paper it is referred to as "hard copy," inferring that it can be handled and carried from the area.

33. *d.* Military or 24-hour time is used on computer-generated labels. The specimen should be collected at 1400 hours or 2 PM.

34. *b.* The specimen code on the label is 1-blue, which indicates one blue top or sodium citrate tube

35. *a.* A patient's identification number may be a health care facility generated number or social security number.

Laboratory Math

16

REVIEW QUESTIONS

1. What does 2.2 lb equal in the metric system:
   a. 1 kg
   b. 44 g
   c. 100 g
   d. 454 kg

2. 1.2 kg is equal to how many grams?
   a. 12
   b. 120
   c. 1200
   d. 12,000

3. Body temperature in centigrade degrees is:
   a. 98.6
   b. 37.0
   c. 25.0
   d. 32.0

4. Normal adult blood volume is 70 mL per kilogram. You weigh 130 lb. What is your blood volume?
   a. 1300 mL
   b. 1.3 L

c. 59 kg
d. 4.1 L

5. How is the number 12 written in Roman numerals?
   a. IIV
   b. VII
   c. IIX
   d. XII

6. A test requires 3 mL serum. The laboratory requires that the amount of blood collected be 250% of the volume of specimen required to perform the test. Which size tube should you use to collect the specimen?
   a. 4 mL
   b. 5 mL
   c. 10 mL
   d. 15 mL

7. Your requisition says that a specimen is to be drawn at 1530. What time would that be in 12-hour time?
   a. 1:30 AM
   b. 3:30 PM
   c. 5:30 AM
   d. 7:30 PM

8. The basic unit of volume in the metric system is the:
   a. decimal
   b. gram
   c. liter
   d. meter

9. A blood culture bottle containing 45 mL of media requires a 1:10 dilution of specimen. How much blood should be added?
   a. 4 mL
   b. 5 mL
   c. 8 mL
   d. 10 mL

10. The basic unit of weight in the metric system is the:
    a. gram
    b. liter
    c. meter
    d. ounce

11. To prepare 100 mL of a 1:10 dilution of bleach, add:
    a. 1 mL water to 100 mL bleach
    b. 1 mL bleach to 99 mL water
    c. 10 mL bleach to 90 mL water
    d. 10 mL water to 100 mL bleach

12. If room temperature is 77° F, what is the temperature in centigrade?
    a. 20
    b. 25
    c. 32
    d. 37

13. 10 cc of blood equals approximately:
    a. 1 mL of blood
    b. 5 mL of blood
    c. 10 mL of blood
    d. there is no relationship between cc and mL

14. In the metric system a meter is a measure of:
    a. mass
    b. density
    c. length
    d. volume

15. If a red blood cell is 8 μm in diameter, what is its size in millimeters?
    a. .8
    b. .08
    c. .008
    d. .0008

16. In the metric system the prefix for 1000 is:
    a. centi-
    b. deci-
    c. kilo-
    d. milli-

17. In the metric system, a millimeter is:
    a. 1/10 meter
    b. 1/100 meter
    c. 1/1000 meter
    d. 1/10,000 meter

18. Your text says that factor VIII is the antihemophilic factor. What common Arabic number is this factor?
    a. four
    b. eight

c. thirteen
d. twenty-three

19. Your paper says that you got 45 out of 50 questions correct. What is your grade expressed as a percent?
    a. 45%
    b. 75%
    c. 90%
    d. 95%

20. One teaspoon is approximately:
    a. 1 mL
    b. 5 mL
    c. 10 mL
    d. 15 mL

21. Normal infant blood volume is 100 mL per kilogram. Calculate the approximate blood volume of a baby who weighs 6 lb.
    a. 1.2 L
    b. 2.7 L
    c. 270 mL
    d. 600 mL

22. 1:00 PM in 24-hour time is:
    a. 100
    b. 0100

c. 1300
d. 01300

23. 200 µL is equal to:
    a. 2 mL
    b. 0.2 mL
    c. 0.02 mL
    d. 0.002 mL

24. A specimen must be transported at body temperature, plus or minus 5 degrees Fahrenheit. Which of the following temperature readings is within that range?
    a. 25° Celsius
    b. 35° centigrade
    c. 37° Fahrenheit
    d. 90° Fahrenheit

25. A patient voids 1200 mL of urine for a creatinine clearance test. How much urine is this?
    a. less than a liter
    b. less than a quart
    c. more than a liter
    d. more than two liters

ANSWERS TO REVIEW QUESTIONS

1. **a.** One kilogram equals 2.2 lb (Table 16-1). This is a conversion factor that should be memorized. A helpful hint might be to remember that weight in kilograms is approximately half (divide by 2) the number given in pounds.

2. **c.** To convert metric units from larger units to smaller units move the decimal point to the right the appropriate multiple. A kilogram (Table 16-2) is 1000 or 10^3 g. The multiple, therefore, is 3.

$$1.2 \text{ kg} = 1200 \text{ g.}$$

3. **b.** Body temperature in centigrade is 37 degrees. To calculate body temperature in centigrade when given a Fahrenheit reading, subtract 32 from the Fahrenheit temperature and multiple by 5/9. NOTE: A health care worker should memorize this centigrade temperature along with a few other temperatures which are common when working in health care.

TABLE 16-2. **Commonly Used Measurement Prefixes**

PREFIX	MULTIPLE	Meter	Gram	Liter
		UNIT OF MEASURE		
kilo- (k)	1,000 (10^3)	km	kg	kl
deci- (d)	1/10 (10^{-1})	dm	dg	dl
centi- (c)	1/100 (10^{-2})	cm	cg	cl
milli- (m)	1/1,000 (10^{-3})	mm	mg	ml
micro- (μ)	1/1,000,000 (10^{-6})	μm	μg	μl

4. **d.** Normal adult blood volume is approximately 70 mL per kilogram of weight. If the weight is given in pounds it must be converted to kilograms by multiplying by the conversion factor 0.454 (Table 16-3). The weight in kilograms is multiplied by 70 because we know that for every kilogram of weight in an adult there are 70 mL of blood. Divide the result by 1000 because adult blood volume is reported in liters and 1 L equals 1000 mL.

$$130 \text{ lb} \times 0.454 = 59.02 \text{ kg}$$

$$59 \text{ kg} \times 70 \text{ kg/mL} = 4130 \text{ mL}$$

$$4130/1000 = 4.13 \text{ L}$$

TABLE 16-1. **Metric–English Conversion Equivalents**

	METRIC		ENGLISH
Distance	meter (m)	=	3.3 feet / 39.37 inches
	centimeter (cm)	=	0.4 inches
	millimeter (mm)	=	0.04 inches
Weight	gram (g)	=	.0022 pounds
	kilogram (kg)	=	2.2 pounds
Volume	liter (l)	=	1.06 quarts
	milliliter (ml)	=	.03 fluid ounces
	milliliter (ml)	=	.20 or ⅕ tsp

Note: A milliliter (ml) is approximately equal to a cubic centimeter (cc) and the two terms are often used interchangeably.

TABLE 16-3. **English–Metric Conversion Equivalents**

	ENGLISH		METRIC
Distance	yard (yd)	=	0.9 meters (m)
	inch (in)	=	2.54 centimeters (cm)
Weight	pound (lb)	=	0.454 kilograms (kg) or 454 grams (g)
	ounce (oz)	=	28 grams (g)
Volume	quart (qt)	=	0.95 liters (l)
	fluid ounce (fl oz)	=	30 milliliters (ml)
	tablespoon (tbsp)	=	15 milliliters (ml)
	teaspoon (tsp)	=	5 milliliters (ml)

5. *d.* To write Arabic numbers in Roman numerals, remember the rules. Roman numerals are written from left to right and can never exceed more than three of the same numeral in a sequence. To write the number 12, you should start with a base number such as X = 10 and then add lower value numbers until you reach your desired value, for example, X + I + I = 12.

6. *c.* The laboratory needs 250% or two and one-half times the 3 mL required for the test. Two times 3 mL is 6 mL. One-half of 3 mL is 1 1/2 mL (or you can multiply 3 times 2.5). You need 7 1/2 mL to do the test. The closest correct size tube is 10 mL.

7. *b.* To change 24-hour time to 12-hour time (Fig. 16-1), subtract 1200 from any time after 1300. 1530 in 24-hour time less 1200 is 330 which written in 12-hour time is 3:30 PM.

8. *c.* It is easier to remember that the liter is the basic metric unit of volume than to remember other metric measurements because the "soft drink industry" in the United States has converted much of their packaging to metric measurements and we see advertisements for liters of soft drinks all the time.

9. *b.* A blood culture dilution of 1:10 means there is 1 mL of blood and 9 mL of media for every 10 mL of blood culture specimen. Forty-five milliliters of media is five times the original proportion of 9 mL. To maintain the same 1:10 dilution you must also have five times the original 1 mL proportion of blood. That means you will need to add 5 mL blood to the 45 mL media.

10. *a.* The basic unit of weight in the metric system is the gram.

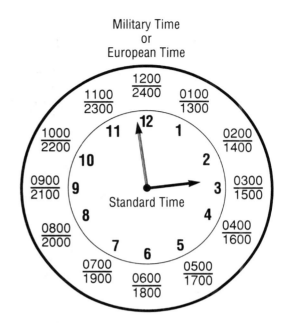

FIGURE 16-1. Clock showing 24-hour (military) time.

11. *c.* A 1:10 dilution of bleach means there is 1 mL of bleach and 9 mL of water for every 10 mL of solution. One hundred milliliters of a 1:10 dilution is 10 times the original 10-mL proportion. That means you will also need 10 times the original amounts of bleach and water; or 10 mL bleach and 90 mL water.

12. *b.* To convert 77° Fahrenheit temperature to centigrade or Celsius (Fig. 16-2), subtract 32 from the Fahrenheit number and multiple the result by 5/9. Health care workers should memorize this commonly referenced centigrade temperature.

$$77 - 32 = 45$$

$$5/9 \, (45) = 5/9 \times 45/1$$

$$5/9 \times 45/1 = 225/9$$

$$225/9 = 25 \text{ degrees centigrade}$$

13. *c.* For practical purposes, *mL* and *cc* are equivalent and the terms are often used interchangeably in a laboratory setting. Both are approximately equal to one-thousandth of a liter. The term *milliliter* is used when referring to liquid volume; *cubic centimeter* is used when referring to volume of gas. However, syringes that are used to extract liquid volume are often calibrated in cc rather than mL.

14. *c.* The metric measurement for length is meter (m).

15. *c.* A micrometer (or micron) (Table 16-3) is equal to one-millionth of a meter and a millimeter is equal to one-thousandth of a meter which means you are converting smaller units to larger units. To do this, the decimal point moves to the left the same number of times as the multiple to which you are converting. A millimeter is 10^{-3} m. The multiple is three, so the decimal point moves three places to the left.

$$008.0 \; \gamma m = .008 \; mL$$

16. *c.* Kilo- abbreviated "k" means 1000. It can be used with each of the three basic units of measure in the metric system.

kilogram (kg) = 1000 grams (g)

kiloliter (kL) = 1000 liters (L)

kilometer (km) = 1000 meters (m)

17. *c.* A millimeter is 1/1000 meter or 10^{-3} m.

18. *b.* If V = 5 and I = 1, than VIII is 5 + 1 + 1 + 1 or 8.

19. *c.* To calculate a percentage, a number must be converted to parts per 100. First make the number a fraction. Then multiply the numerator of the fraction by 100, divide by the denominator, and add a percent sign.

$$45/50 \times 100 = 45/50 \times 100/1$$
$$= 4500/50 = 90\%$$

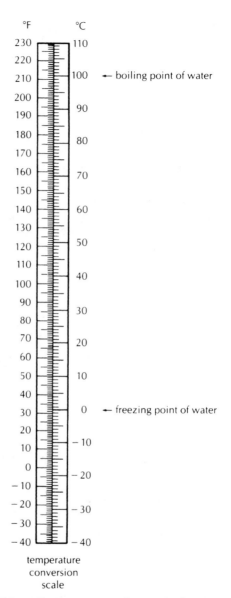

FIGURE 16-2. Thermometer showing both Fahrenheit and Celsius degrees (Memmler RI, Cohen BJ, Wood DL).

20. *b.* By using an English-Metric conversion chart (see Table 16–3), you can find the right answer or you may choose to memorize certain common conversions, such as 1 tsp = 5 mL.

21. *c.* Normal infant blood volume is approximately 100 mL/kg. If a baby's weight is given in pounds, it must be converted to kilograms by multiplying the pounds by the conversion factor 0.454. Once the weight is established in kilograms, multiply that number by 100 because for every kilogram there are 100 mL of blood.

6 lb $\times$ 0.454 = 2.7 kg (rounded to nearest tenth)

2.7 kg $\times$ 100 mL/kg = 270 mL or .27 L

22. *c.* To convert 12-hour time to 24-hour time, add 1200 to the time from 1 PM on; 1:00 without the colon is 100. 100 plus 1200 becomes 1300.

23. *b.* Microliters are smaller units than milliliters. In the metric system it is possible to convert a smaller unit to a larger unit by moving the decimal point to the left by the amount of the multiple of the unit you are converting to. One milliliter equals one-thousandth of a liter or 10^{-3} liters. The multiple is minus three. Therefore, to convert 200 microliters to milliliters, move the decimal point three places to the left.

200.0 = .2 mL

24. *b.* Fahrenheit body temperature is 98.6°. Once we add and subtract 5; we know that we are looking for a temperature that is between 93.6° F and 103.6° F. This eliminates 37° F and 90° F. Celsius and centigrade are the same; 25° Celsius is the same as 77° F. The remaining choice is 35° C. To convert 35° C to Fahrenheit temperature:

(9/5 $\times$ 35) + 32 = 63 + 32 = 95° F.

25. *c.* A liter is equal to 1000 mL and a quart is equal to 950 mL; therefore 1200 mL is 200 mL more than a liter and 250 mL more than a quart and 800 mL less than 2 L.

Comprehensive Mock Exam

II

EXAM QUESTIONS

1. The physician requests a serum sample for a special test to be sent out. Which of the following tubes should be used?
   a. green top
   b. lavender top
   c. light blue top
   d. red top

2. The hospital program that does scheduled audits to review patient care is called:
   a. outpatient services
   b. patient care
   c. quality assurance
   d. support services

3. The patient must void the last sample of a 24-hour urine collection:
   a. at exactly the time the collection is ended
   b. immediately after dinner that day
   c. one hour before the test is over
   d. whenever his/her bladder is full

4. A person who has 2 years of education and performs laboratory testing, maintains quality control, and works independently is a:
   a. Clinical Laboratory Technician
   b. Medical Technologist
   c. Pathologist
   d. Specimen Processor

5. Inflammation of a vein is called:
   a. arteriosclerosis
   b. cellulitis
   c. phlebitis
   d. thrombosis

6. After the preferred median cubital vein, the next choice for venipuncture is:
   a. basilic vein
   b. cephalic vein
   c. dorsal hand vein
   d. ulnar vein

7. Causative agents in the "Chain of Infection" are all of the following except:
   a. bacteria
   b. parasites
   c. patients
   d. viruses

8. Patients must be fasting for all of the following tests except:
   a. cholesterol
   b. cortisol
   c. glucose
   d. triglycerides

9. Aerosols can be produced by:
   a. centrifuging open serum tubes
   b. popping open blood containers
   c. pouring off a serum sample
   d. all of the above

10. Massaging the forearm from elbow to wrist, heat application on the area, and palpitating at the vein site all aid in:
    a. avoiding hemolyzing the specimen
    b. decreasing vascular distention
    c. increasing peripheral dilation of the vein
    d. preventing the formation of a hematoma

11. Which of the following techniques should be used when performing skin punctures?
    a. long-tip lancet should be used for optimum blood collection
    b. strong, repetitive pressure should be applied
    c. use povidone iodine to cleanse the skin surface
    d. wipe away the first drop of blood that forms

12. Which of the following additives is used to speed up clotting?
    a. citrate
    b. EDTA
    c. oxalate
    d. thrombin

13. The only diagnostic test listed below that the patient must be fasting for is:
    a. APPT
    b. disseminated intravascular coagulation (DIC) screen

c. prothrombin time
d. triglycerides

14. The preferred method of transportation for laboratory specimens from isolation rooms is:
    a. double-bagging with brown paper bags
    b. double-bagging with clear plastic bags
    c. placement in paper cups marked "warning"
    d. washing specimen container with alcohol

15. "Blood and body fluid precautions consistently used for all patients regardless of their bloodborne infection status" is the definition of:
    a. Infection Control
    b. Isolation Techniques
    c. Protective Procedures
    d. Universal Precautions

16. "Universal Precautions" recommends all of the following except:
    a. dismissal of HIV-positive workers
    b. frequent handwashing
    c. HBV immunization
    d. use of protective barriers

17. The test(s) used to provide information about the patient's acid–base balance is/are:
    a. ABG
    b. BUN
    c. LDH
    d. Na & K

18. An antiseptic is a chemical agent that will:
    a. inhibit the growth of microorganisms
    b. interfere with the test that is to be performed
    c. stop the growth of microorganisms
    d. usually cause a reaction in the patient

19. The precentrifugation time for a serum separator tube is:
    a. 5 minutes
    b. 10 minutes
    c. 15 minutes
    d. 30 minutes

20. All of the following are examples of antiseptics except:
    a. alcohol
    b. hydrogen peroxide
    c. phenol
    d. tincture of iodine

21. Which of the following instruments is usually located in a central processing area of the laboratory?
    a. blood gas analyzer
    b. centrifuge
    c. chemistry analyzer
    d. all of the above

22. Exposure to HIV and HBV can be prevented by the use of appropriate barriers. For a phlebotomist performing a routine venipuncture, the barrier indicated is:
    a. gloves
    b. gown
    c. mask
    d. plastic apron

23. The first action a phlebotomist should take when a hematoma begins to form while performing venipuncture is:
    a. apply ice above the area
    b. apply pressure to the area
    c. remove the needle
    d. remove the tourniquet

24. Class "C" fires involve which of the following materials:
    a. combustible metals
    b. electrical equipment
    c. paper
    d. wood

25. The antiseptic of choice for collecting ETOH levels is:
    a. 70% isopropyl alcohol
    b. 70% methyl alcohol
    c. distilled water
    d. hexachlorophene

26. The smallest needle lumen listed below is:
    a. 18 gauge
    b. 21 gauge

    c. 23 gauge
    d. 25 gauge

27. The most commonly used, easily accessible artery used for blood gas sampling is the:
    a. brachial artery
    b. femoral artery
    c. radial artery
    d. ulnar artery

28. A pregnant phlebotomist has been requested to draw blood from a patient with rubella. She should do the following:
    a. ask the floor nurse to accompany her into the room
    b. draw the patient using respiratory isolation precautions
    c. request another phlebotomist to draw the patient
    d. use strict isolation precautions to draw the patient

29. Which additive is used to keep glucose values stable in plasma?
    a. ammonium oxalate
    b. sodium citrate
    c. potassium oxalate
    d. sodium fluoride

30. Symptoms of shock include all of the following *except*:
    a. moist, clammy skin
    b. expressionless stare
    c. severe thirst
    d. weak, rapid pulse

31. Capillary blood gas equipment includes all of the following *except:*
    a. flea & magnet
    b. lancet
    c. Natelson collection tube
    d. syringe & butterfly

32. If a tourniquet is left on too long it can cause:
    a. hemoconcentration
    b. discomfort to the patient
    c. erroneous lab results
    d. all of the above

33. The sagittal plane divides the body:
    a. into right and left halves
    b. into upper and lower sections
    c. lengthwise from side to side
    d. none of the above

34. Blood returns to the heart from the lungs into the:
    a. left atrium
    b. left ventricle
    c. right atrium
    d. right ventricle

35. What layer of the arterial vessel is markedly different from that of the vein?
    a. endothelium
    b. connective tissue
    c. internal elastic lamina
    d. smooth muscle

36. The "Chain of Infection" involves all of these steps except:
    a. causative agents
    b. infection control
    c. means of transmission
    d. susceptible host

37. The physician has requested a CBC and cardiac enzymes. Which tubes should you use to collect the specimen?
    a. blue and lavender tubes
    b. green and red tubes
    c. red and blue tubes
    d. red and lavender tubes

38. Which of the following test results is *not* falsely elevated by Betadine contamination?
    a. bilirubin
    b. hemoglobin
    c. potassium
    d. uric acid

39. The purpose in warming the heel of an infant for capillary blood gas analysis is to:
    a. arterialize the sample
    b. collect a warm sample
    c. make the infant more comfortable
    d. prevent hematomas

40. The sweat chloride test is used in the diagnosis of:
    a. cystic fibrosis
    b. enzyme deficiency
    c. pancreatitis
    d. stress

41. "Susceptible hosts" to infection are those people who:
    a. eat in the hospital cafeteria
    b. lack resistance to infection
    c. visit the hospital
    d. work closely with patients

42. After drug administration, the peak level is usually determined and blood drawn at:
    a. 10 minutes
    b. 30 minutes
    c. 90 minutes
    d. 120 minutes

43. The Allen Test should be performed before an arterial puncture:
    a. to assess circulation
    b. to improve circulation
    c. to warm the hand
    d. all of the above

44. Bleeding times are performed most often:
    a. after surgery
    b. during surgery
    c. never on surgical patients
    d. prior to surgery

45. In cleansing the phlebotomy site for a blood culture, the pad with the antiseptic is moved in the following manner:
    a. back and forth, across the site several times
    b. in a circular motion, from the center outward
    c. in a circular motion, from the periphery inward
    d. up and down, starting at the top

46. The purpose of protective isolation is to:
    a. prevent airborne transmission of disease
    b. protect the patient from outside contamination
    c. protect the hospital employee from patients' diseases
    d. provide a safe environment for pediatric patients

47. The single most important means of preventing the spread of infection is:
    a. handwashing before and after contact with each patient
    b. identifying the disease being isolated
    c. wearing gloves when drawing blood from an infectious patient
    d. wearing a mask into isolation rooms

48. The part of the needle that is measured in inches is called the:
    a. bevel
    b. hub
    c. lumen
    d. shaft

49. It is necessary to control the depth of lancet insertion during skin puncture to avoid:
    a. bacterial contamination
    b. bone penetration
    c. excessive bleeding
    d. puncturing a vein

50. The proper angle of the spreader slide, when preparing a slide wedge smear, should be approximately:
    a. 15 degrees
    b. 30 degrees
    c. 60 degrees
    d. 90 degrees

51. The effect anchoring the vein has on venipuncture is:
    a. it causes hemoconcentration
    b. it increases localized blood flow
    c. it keeps veins from rolling
    d. it makes veins stand out

52. A physician suspects that a child has pertussis and orders a nasopharyngeal culture. What site is swabbed in order to obtain a proper specimen as requested?

a. back of the throat
b. inside the nose beyond the nares
c. the inner ear
d. where pus is present

53. Specimens can be rejected because of:
   a. discrepancy between the requisition and label
   b. unlabeled tubes
   c. both of the above
   d. neither of the above

54. What standard requires manufacturers to supply MSDS information for hazardous materials?
   a. Bloodborne Pathogen Standard
   b. CDC Universal Precautions
   c. HAZCOM Standards
   d. NCCLS M29T

55. Why is the proper antiseptic especially important in blood culture collection?
   a. more bacteria are present on the skin of patients with suspected septicemia
   b. pathogenic bacteria will not grow in media if the wrong antiseptic is used
   c. the wrong antiseptic may cause serious complications to the patient
   d. there is a significant risk of blood culture contamination from bacteria on the skin

56. As many as six items may be included on the "receipt labels" for fluids other than blood delivered to the lab. In addition to the patient name and number, what other item must be included:
   a. doctor ordering
   b. room number
   c. specimen type
   d. test ordered

57. An unconscious, unidentified man is admitted to an emergency trauma center. What would be the system of choice to ensure patient identification?
   a. assign a name to the patient, such as John Doe, and utilize that name for identification
   b. assign a number to the patient until the patient can be identified
   c. use a three-part identification system that utilizes a temporary armband and labels for specimens and blood to be transfused
   d. wait to process any samples until the patient can be identified

58. Class B fires occur:
   a. in or near electrical equipment
   b. with combustible materials like wood
   c. with combustible metals
   d. with flammable liquids

59. Skin punctures should be made:
   a. parallel to the fingerprints
   b. perpendicular to the fingerprints
   c. where there are no fingerprints
   d. none of the above

60. Which of the following is an anticoagulant?
   a. citrate
   b. glass particles
   c. thixotropic gel
   d. thrombin

61. A tourniquet should be left on no longer than:
   a. two minutes
   b. sixty seconds
   c. the time it takes to gather all of your equipment
   d. the time it takes to get the needle seated in the vein

62. Which part of a syringe is calibrated?
   a. adapter
   b. barrel
   c. hub
   d. plunger

63. Which of the following is not true of a vacutainer needle?
   a. it has dual points
   b. it comes in different lengths
   c. it is reusable
   d. it is sterile

64. Which of the following would be the antiseptic(s) of choice for blood culture collection?
    a. 0.5% chlorhexidine gluconate
    b. 70% isopropyl alcohol
    c. 1% to 2% tincture of iodine
    d. use of both 70% isopropyl alcohol and 1% to 2% tincture of iodine

65. The agency responsible for investigating communicable diseases is:
    a. AMA
    b. CDC
    c. JCAHO
    d. OSHA

66. The capillary container that has color-coded caps for identifying specific additives is called:
    a. autolet
    b. hematocrit tubes
    c. microtainer
    d. Natelson tubes

67. The ratio of compressions to ventilations for one-person CPR on an adult is:
    a. 5 to 1
    b. 10 to 2
    c. 15 to 1
    d. 15 to 2

68. Approximately 10 cc of blood is drawn for electrolytes, CBC, and PT using a syringe. What is the proper order in which to fill the evacuated tubes from the syringe?
    a. blue, red, lavender
    b. blue, lavender, red
    c. lavender, blue, red
    d. red, blue, lavender

69. The green-capped tube contains:
    a. ethylenediaminetetraacetate
    b. potassium oxalate
    c. sodium citrate
    d. sodium heparin

70. An example of an enteric isolation disease is:
    a. hepatitis
    b. measles
    c. meningitis
    d. tuberculosis

71. When someone becomes a victim of electrical shock, the first step to take is:
    a. call an ambulance
    b. give breathing aid
    c. give CPR
    d. shut off power source

72. A naturally occurring anticoagulant is:
    a. citrate
    b. EDTA
    c. heparin
    d. thrombin

73. Thixotropic gel is a/an:
    a. antibacterial agent
    b. anticoagulant
    c. red-cell preservative
    d. serum separator

74. The part of the needle that has angled cuts for ease of insertion is called:
    a. bevel
    b. hub
    c. lumen
    d. shaft

75. The department in the laboratory that provides units of blood for transfusions is:
    a. coagulation
    b. hematology
    c. immunohematology
    d. phlebotomy

76. Which specimen should be protected from light?
    a. ammonia
    b. bilirubin
    c. phosphorus
    d. potassium

77. In order to use the hospital computer correctly, the user must be able to:
    a. repair any mechanical malfunctions
    b. recognize the proper commands for execution

c. type at least 50 words per minute on the computer keyboard

d. understand the programming of the computer

78. Which information is not required on an inpatient specimen requisition?
    a. patient full name
    b. physician name
    c. patient date of birth
    d. physician's address

79. Special precautions for specimens placed in pneumatic tube systems include those for:
    a. leak protection
    b. separation of specimens to prevent breakage
    c. shock protection
    d. all of the above

80. When shipping biological specimens to another laboratory, which is not a recommended procedure?
    a. affix address or telephone number of CDC
    b. indicate on label if dry ice is used
    c. label as biohazardous medical specimen
    d. label specimen from AIDS patient "HIV"

81. Urine for culture should be transported in what manner?
    a. at 37°C as soon as possible
    b. at room temperature, within one hour
    c. at room temperature, within 2 to 3 hours
    d. on ice, as soon as possible

82. "Nosocomial" is an infection:
    a. found in public places
    b. found only in the intensive care unit
    c. that is hospital acquired
    d. brought to patients by visitors

83. When blood is collected from a patient, the serum should be separated from the blood cells as quickly as possible to avoid:

a. glycolysis
b. hemoconcentration
c. hemolysis
d. hemostasis

84. When a fire occurs, the first thing that should be done is:
    a. call the number assigned
    b. contain the fire yourself
    c. evacuate the area
    d. pull the alarm box nearest you

85. A tachometer is an instrument that determines the:
    a. concentration of cholesterol in a blood drop
    b. correct pressure of a blood pressure cuff
    c. glucose level of a sample
    d. revolution per minute of a centrifuge

86. All of the following are examples of disinfectants except:
    a. alcohol
    b. formaldehyde
    c. hypochlorite solution
    d. phenol

87. Chemicals used to remove or kill pathogenic microbes on inanimate surfaces are called:
    a. analgesics
    b. anesthetics
    c. antiseptics
    d. disinfectants

88. A physician has requested that a CBC and electrolytes be performed on her patient. You cannot draw blood by venipuncture; you have to perform a fingerstick. What should you collect first?
    a. purple top microtainer
    b. red top microtainer
    c. smear for differential
    d. two hematocrit tubes

89. Blood specimens should not be drawn from the side of a patient on which a mastectomy was performed because of:

    a. edema in tissue
    b. hemolysis
    c. lymphostasis
    d. pain in the arm

90. In a skin puncture procedure, hemolysis may occur due to:
    a. heat application to site
    b. a lancet that is too long
    c. squeezing the heel or finger too hard
    d. tissue fluid contamination

91. Indwelling lines may be inserted into a patient for the purpose of collecting diagnostic blood specimens and for fluid and medication administration. The risks associated with obtaining blood from these lines are the tendency to develop thrombosis and:
    a. a hematoma
    b. hemolysis of the sample
    c. infection at the line site
    d. infiltration into tissue

92. A diabetic patient has an IV line in her right hand. She also has an IV line in her left arm halfway between her wrist and the antecubital fossa. Her leg veins are inaccessible and all of her fingers are grossly edematous. The physician orders a STAT glucose and CBC. What do you do?
    a. collect the specimen by fingerstick
    b. inform the nurse that a phlebotomy cannot be done on this patient
    c. perform the venipuncture using a vein in her left hand
    d. perform the venipuncture using a vein in her right antecubital fossa area

93. The first step when entering an isolation room is to:
    a. assemble the equipment needed
    b. put on a gown
    c. read the sign on the door to determine the type of isolation
    d. wash the hands

94. A(n) _____ is a medical doctor who treats female reproductive tract disorders.
    a. cardiologist
    b. endocrinologist
    c. orthopedist
    d. gynecologist

95. A blood alcohol level is ordered STAT by the ER physician. You begin the venipuncture procedure by using an alcohol-soaked gauze pad to wipe the site. Immediately you realize what you have done. What is your next step?
    a. be sure that the alcohol has completely evaporated from the skin and then continue the phlebotomy
    b. continue the phlebotomy but note on the test request that you had used alcohol for cleansing the site
    c. discontinue the phlebotomy and notify the nurse that you have contaminated the patient with an outside source of alcohol
    d. discontinue the venipuncture; perform the phlebotomy on the other arm using Betadine instead to cleanse the site

96. Gel separator tubes should not be used for:
    a. blood bank specimens
    b. chemistry specimens
    c. drug level specimens
    d. glucose tolerance tests

97. Specimens used in glucose tolerance tests and therapeutic drug monitoring have which of the following collection requirements?
    a. must be taken while patient is fasting
    b. must be iced
    c. must be taken by skin puncture only
    d. collection must be timed

98. In communicating information to a patient so that a specimen can be collected, the best method for

determining whether the patient understood the information would be to:

a. ask the patient to repeat information
b. assume the patient understood
c. ask the patient to read a specimen collection sheet
d. repeat the information a second time

99. Some barriers or filters that block patient understanding of information might be:

a. cultural differences
b. emotions such as anger, fear, and distrust
c. a handicap such as deafness
d. all of the above

100. Breach of confidentiality is:

a. failure to exercise a reasonable amount of care
b. identification of a risk without reporting it
c. touching a person without their consent
d. unauthorized release of information concerning a patient

Appendix

ANSWERS TO
COMPREHENSIVE MOCK EXAM

1.	*d*	26.	*d*	51.	*c*	76.	*b*
2.	*c*	27.	*c*	52.	*b*	77.	*b*
3.	*a*	28.	*c*	53.	*c*	78.	*d*
4.	*a*	29.	*d*	54.	*c*	79.	*d*
5.	*c*	30.	*c*	55.	*d*	80.	*d*
6.	*b*	31.	*d*	56.	*c*	81.	*b*
7.	*c*	32.	*d*	57.	*c*	82.	*c*
8.	*b*	33.	*a*	58.	*d*	83.	*a*
9.	*d*	34.	*a*	59.	*b*	84.	*d*
10.	*c*	35.	*d*	60.	*a*	85.	*d*
11.	*d*	36.	*b*	61.	*b*	86.	*a*
12.	*d*	37.	*d*	62.	*b*	87.	*d*
13.	*d*	38.	*b*	63.	*c*	88.	*c*
14.	*b*	39.	*a*	64.	*d*	89.	*c*
15.	*d*	40.	*a*	65.	*b*	90.	*c*
16.	*a*	41.	*b*	66.	*c*	91.	*c*
17.	*a*	42.	*b*	67.	*d*	92.	*c*
18.	*a*	43.	*a*	68.	*b*	93.	*c*
19.	*c*	44.	*d*	69.	*d*	94.	*d*
20.	*c*	45.	*b*	70.	*a*	95.	*d*
21.	*b*	46.	*b*	71.	*d*	96.	*a*
22.	*a*	47.	*d*	72.	*c*	97.	*d*
23.	*d*	48.	*d*	73.	*d*	98.	*a*
24.	*b*	49.	*b*	74.	*a*	99.	*d*
25.	*d*	50.	*b*	75.	*c*	100.	*d*

INDEX

Page numbers followed by *f* indicate illustrations;
t following a page number indicates tabular material.